STUDENT LEARNING

for

Beare/Myers *Adult Health Nursing*

THIRD EDITION

Prepared by

Golden M. Tradewell, MSN, MA, RN

Assistant Professor
College of Nursing
McNeese State University
Lake Charles, Louisiana

Acknowledgements for past contributors:

Carole A. Broxon, RN, PhD
Carolyn A. Patiño, RN, MSN
Donita T. Qualey, RN, MN

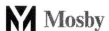 Mosby

St. Louis Baltimore Boston Carlsbad Chicago Minneapolis New York Philadelphia Portland
London Milan Sydney Tokyo Toronto

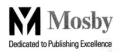

Mosby
Dedicated to Publishing Excellence

A Times Mirror
Company

Publisher   Sally Schrefer
Editor   Michael S. Ledbetter
Associate Developmental Editor   Kristin Geen
Project Manager   Gayle Morris
Manufacturing Manager   Betty Mueller
Design and Layout   DocuComp Services
Cover Design   Amy Buxton

Mosby–Year Book, Inc.
11830 Westline Industrial Drive
St. Louis, Missouri 63146
International Standard Book Number 0-8151-1012-X
29579

97 98 99 00 01 / 9 8 7 6 5 4 3 2 1

Table of Contents

Critical
Thinking
Worksheets

Critical Thinking Worksheet

Name _____

 CHAPTER *1* **Infection**

1. Locate the charts of three patients who have infections. Compare and contrast among those patients:
   a. Chief complaint that led to health care
      1.

      2.

      3.

   b. Medical diagnosis
      1.

      2.

      3.

   c. Signs and symptoms of infection
      1.

      2.

      3.

Continued

1

d. Causative organism source
   1.

   2.

   3.

e. Antibiotic sensitivity (lab report)
   1.

   2.

   3.

f. Antibiotics administered
   1.

   2.

   3.

g. Effectiveness of antibiotics
   1.

Continued

2.

3.

h. Side effects
    1.

    2.

    3.

i. Dosage/route
    1.

    2.

    3.

j. Nonmedication intervention for infection
    1.

    2.

    3.

Continued

2. List the signs and symptoms of infection.

3. Describe how signs and symptoms of infection in the immune depressed and the elderly may differ from those of the adult.

Critical Thinking Worksheet   Name _____

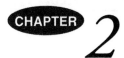 **CHAPTER** *2*   **Fluids, Electrolytes, and Acid-Base Balance**

1. A dehydrated patient produces very small amounts of concentrated urine. What physiologic processes are responsible for this type of urinary output?

2. Elicit and describe the clinical significance of the following:
   a. Trousseau's sign

   b. Chvostek's sign

3. List and describe three laboratory tests that would be useful in assessing electrolyte imbalance.

4. You become ill with the "stomach flu." You are feverish, perspiring, and experiencing severe nausea and vomiting. What fluid and electrolyte imbalance might you be at risk of developing?

5. What relationship exists between the chloride shift and the oxyhemoglobin curve?

6. Explain how various clinical situations may cause acid-base disturbance. Suggest ABG values that would be consistent with:

	PaCO$_2$	pH	HCO$_3$
Compensated metabolic alkalosis			
Early hyperventilation			
Uncompensated metabolic alkalosis			

7. Complete the following chart:

Electrolyte and Normal Value	Main Functions	Clinical Manifestations of Excess	Clinical Manifestations of Deficit
Sodium:			
Potassium:			
Calcium:			
Magnesium:			

8. Fill a pitcher with 1 liter of water; weigh it, pour out the water, and weigh the empty pitcher. Subtract the weight of the pitcher from the total. Now, recall a patient you recently cared for who was receiving IV fluids. Recalling that patient's IV rate, how many pounds/ounces of fluid did he/she receive in 24 hours? 72 hours? How significant is this for the patient with heart disease? renal disease? normal aging? How does the intake relate to fluid loss from the body?

9. Your patient was admitted with respiratory acidosis secondary to his emphysema. His wife asks you, "Will I need to do blood sugars on John for his acidosis like I do for my diabetic acidosis?"
   a. List the pathophysiological concepts which need to be taught.

   b. Develop a teaching plan for this family.

10. The physician orders insulin and hypertonic IV dextrose for the non-diabetic patient whose serum potassium level is 5.7 mEq/L. State your rationale for following this order.

Critical Thinking Worksheet

Name _____

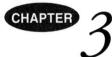 Pain

1. Develop a care plan for a patient experiencing postoperative pain, including diagnoses, expected outcomes, and interventions appropriate to the acute experience. Include alternative therapies to pain medication.

2. Determine which medications are most commonly used in your current clinical setting. For each of these medications, write the generic and trade names, usual adult dosage range, usual side effects, and nursing actions associated with the drug's administration.

3. Identify which type of pain is being described below, choosing from these terms: acute, chronic, referred, visceral, and central.
   a. Deep, difficult to localize: _____

   b. Perceived away from the source: _____

   c. Reversible, specific, short duration: _____

   d. Intense, burning, difficult to control: _____

   e. Begins gradually, persists: _____

4. A patient with a fractured knee cap requests that his opioid be injected directly into his knee, "because that's where it hurts." Develop a teaching explanation, based on the pathophysiology of pain transmission and the analgesic action of opiates, for this patient.

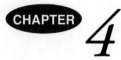

CHAPTER

4 Neoplasia

1. Complete the following chart:

Agent	Therapeutic Action	Toxic Effects	Nursing Activities Associated with Administration
Radiation			
Chemotherapy			

2. A nurse is assigned to a patient with cancer who is in reverse isolation. The nurse, who has a cold, is just about to enter the patient's room. Should she do so? What actions might you take? Why?

3. In your clinical setting, identify environmental carcinogens, if present, and list below.

4. What measures can you take to control or minimize pain in your patient with cancer?

Continued

5. In patients with cancer, identify the physiologic basis for each of the following:
   a. Pain

   b. Bleeding

   c. Infection

   d. Alopecia

6. Your patient was told just now that she has breast cancer, and the oncologist recommended a modified mastectomy with follow-up chemotherapy. She is sobbing and tells you, "My husband can't handle this. He'll leave me if I have my breast removed." Discuss your response and which resources you will consult for this patient.

7. A patient with testicular cancer tested positive for the tumor marker Alpha-fetoprotein. Following surgery and chemotherapy, he tested negative and was told he was in "remission." Two years later, during a routine exam, the oncologist told the patient the marker was positive and he would be started on chemo again. The patient said, "I don't understand. I feel great!" Explain tumor markers for this patient.

8. Your patient is receiving radiation therapy for ovarian cancer. Discuss nursing measures you would implement for the following:
   a. Itching, sore, dry skin

   b. Skin "markings" drawn on lower abdomen

   c. Foul smelling, brown vaginal discharge

   d. Nausea and anorexia

   e. Weight loss of 8 lb. in 1 week

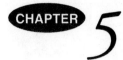 **Shock**

1. Outline usual findings for each stage of shock.

Parameter	Initial Stage	Compensatory Stage	Progressive Stage	Refractory Stage
Level of consciousness				
Skin				
Urine output				
Blood pressure				
Pulse				

2. Consider, individually, three patients for whom you have cared. Were these patients at risk for shock? Why or why not? If at risk, what type of shock would each patient have experienced?

Continued

3. As shock progresses and compensatory mechanisms fail, changes occur. Indicate those changes (e.g., increase or decrease) and the rational in regard to:

	Change	Rationale
Heart rate		
Heart rhythm		
Blood pressure		
Pulse pressure		
Peripheral pulses		
Skin color		
Skin temperature		
Respiratory rate		
Respiratory depth		
Breath sounds		
Bowel sounds		

4. A patient experiences anaphylactic shock secondary to a penicillin injection. State the rationale for each of the following interventions:

Medication	Rationale
Epinephrine	
Antihistamines	
Steroids	

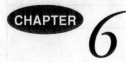

The Critically Ill Adult with Multiple Organ
Dysfunction Syndrome

1. Define multiple organ dysfunction syndrome (MODS).

2. Explain MODS in terms of:
   a. Etiology

   b. Epidemiology

   c. Clinical manifestations
      1. Cardiovascular

      2. Pulmonary

Continued

3. Gastrointestinal

4. Central nervous

5. Renal

6. Hematologic

d. Treatments (medical and nursing)
   1. Oxygen

   2. Nutrition

   3. Organ support

   4. Psychologic support

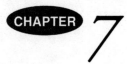

CHAPTER 7   Preoperative Nursing

1. How does patient teaching differ for ambulatory surgery versus inpatient surgery?

2. Explain the significance of abnormal laboratory findings for each of these commonly performed preoperative laboratory tests.
   a. Hemoglobin

   b. Hematocrit

   c. White blood cell count (WBC)

   d. Platelets

   e. Urinalysis
      1. Appearance

      2. Color

      3. Specific gravity

Continued

3. Name two intravenous solutions that are commonly administered during surgery. What are the main constituents of these solutions, and why, specifically, is each administered?

4. Older adults generally take longer to prepare for surgery and longer to recover from surgery. List which factors are slowed and the rationale for that (example given below).

Factor	Rationale
Preop teaching	Learning takes longer; hearing and vision are diminished; language is technical

5. Spend one clinical day with a Certified Registered Nurse Anesthetist (CRNA). Observe the CRNA and discuss:
   a. Necessary preoperative assessment

   b. Necessary postoperative assessment

   c. The decision regarding appropriate anesthetic agents for a specific patient

   d. Measures to ensure patient safety

Critical Thinking Worksheet

Name _____

 CHAPTER **8** **Intraoperative Nursing**

1. Define the term *balanced anesthesia.*

2. What are the advantages of balanced anesthesia?

3. Although factors such as severe pain and hemorrhage affect vital signs, anesthetic agents also affect blood pressure, temperature, pulse, and respiration. In the following chart, indicate the specific effects of selected agents on vital signs:

Drug	Effect on Blood Pressure	Effect on Pulse	Effect on Respiration	Effect on Body Temperature
Thiopental				
Etomidate				
Halothane				
Penthrane				
Ketamine				

Continued

4. Explain complications associated with at least three dangers of improper surgical positioning.

5. Develop a teaching guide for a patient who will have spinal anesthesia. State your rationale for the content of the teaching guide.

Content	Rationale

6. Develop a teaching plan for the spouse of a patient who was diagnosed with "malignant hyperthermia."

7. Return to the skills lab and practice aseptic hand washing and surgical hand washing. List how the procedures differ and the rationale for those differences.

Difference	Rationale

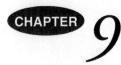

CHAPTER *9*   **Postoperative Nursing**

1. Name at least two analgesics commonly used postoperatively that may produce respiratory depression.

2. A postoperative patient experiences persistent hiccoughs. What interventions and therapeutic measures may be necessary with this patient?

3. Why does obesity contribute to dehiscence?

4. A patient is receiving full fluids. Name foods that would be good sources of the following nutrients for this patient:
   a. Proteins

   b. Ascorbic acid

   c. Vitamin A

   d. Vitamin D

   e. Zinc

Continued

5. Develop a nurse-to-nurse report on a hypothetical patient who is ready to be transferred out of PACU after a thyroidectomy.

6. Observe five surgical and five nonsurgical (decubiti, trauma, etc.) wounds in the clinical agency. Narratively chart or document each wound as explicitly as possible.

7. Perform wound care on the patient on your unit with the most complicated wound. Narratively document the wound and your nursing actions.

CHAPTER *10*   **Nursing Assessment of the Respiratory System**

1. Why must respiratory assessment be complete for a surgical patient both before and after surgery?

2. A patient who is severely dypneic and cyanotic is brought in to the emergency department. What assessments would you make at this time? Why?

3. Develop a set of questions that you might use in a health history to assess respiratory function.

4. Go to the hospital library or the nursing school skills laboratory and review the videotape on breath sounds.

5. Ask the nursing staff which patients have abnormal breath sounds. With permission of each patient, listen to his or her breath sounds.

6. Ask the nurses to help you find a patient who is on a ventilator. With that patient's or family's permission, listen to his or her breath sounds.

7. Locate a patient who has COPD and, with his or her permission, perform a respiratory assessment.

Continued

8. Arrange to observe the technician who performs pulmonary function studies. Define the specific tests performed and their significance.

Test	Significance

CHAPTER

11   **Nursing Interventions Common to Respiratory Disorders**

1. Indicate the positioning that should be used if you are draining the:
   a. Left and right upper lobe anterior apical bronchi

   b. Right middle lobe bronchus

   c. Left lower lobe lateral bronchus

   d. Left and right posterior basal bronchi

2. What safety precautions must the nurse observe during the administration of oxygen?

3. Describe nursing interventions that are associated with aerosol therapy.

Continued

4. What is the essential difference between PEEP and CMV?

5. Develop a nursing care plan for a patient with a chest tube.

6. Develop a teaching response for the patient with pneumonia who refuses to use his incentive spirometer and says, "That's a stupid looking little toy. It can't possibly help my lungs."

7. Spend a clinical day in the Intensive Care Unit. Observe and assist the nurse in performing:
   a. Nasotracheal suction
   b. Tracheostomy/endotracheal tube suctioning
   c. Tracheostomy care
   d. Care of patients on ventilators
   e. Mouth care on unconscious patients

8. Develop a plan for potential emergencies with the ventilator-dependent patient by completing the following statements.
   a. If the endotracheal tube/trach were accidentally pulled out, I would. . .

Continued

b. If the ventilator alarm sounded, I would. . .

c. If the ventilator tubing filled with condensation, I would. . .

d. If the ventilator tubing became disconnected from the trach/endotrach tube, I would. . .

e. If the patient were in distress and the ventilator alarm were sounding and I didn't know what is wrong, I would. . .

CHAPTER *12*   **Nursing Management of Adults with Upper Airway Disorders**

1. Is a support group available in your region for patients with laryngectomies?

2. As a nurse, how could you connect your postoperative laryngectomy patient with this group? (Describe the referral process, and list contact persons.)

3. Research and summarize the speech therapies that a postlaryngectomy patient must receive.

13 Nursing Management of Adults with Lower Airway Disorders

1. You encounter a car accident. A single individual is conscious and supine on the pavement. What signs and symptoms would lead you to suspect a sucking chest wound, and what would you do if he did have this problem?

2. Develop a nursing care plan for a patient with acute ventilatory failure. Include nursing diagnoses, expected outcomes, interventions, and rationales for interventions.

3. Develop a teaching explanation for a 70-year-old male with emphysema who says, "When my breathing gets bad, I'll just turn up my oxygen a little." He is a retired farmer with a sixth grade education who admits that he allows himself ½ cigarette each morning and each evening.

4. How would you most effectively respond to the daughter of your patient with emphysema when she says, "I won't be here when the doctor makes rounds. Please tell him Mother was awake four times last night coughing up that thick stuff. Ask him for some cough medicine so she can sleep tonight."

Continued

5. Compare pneumonia with tuberculosis in regard to:

	Pneumonia	Tuberculosis
Causal organism		
Contributing factors		
Chronic/acute		
Tissue destruction		
Signs/symptoms		
Intervention		

CHAPTER *14*   **Nursing Assessment of the
Peripheral Vascular System**

1. Follow a molecule of glucose from the aorta to the foot and back to the right atrium. Outline the forces that propel the glucose through the system.

2. Draw the location of the temporal, femoral, dorsalis pedis, and posterior tibialis pulses.

3. List the clinical manifestations of an allergic response to contrast medium.

Continued

4. Observe a diagnostic procedure related to the peripheral vascular system. Be sure to include the following:
   a. Perform preprocedure teaching to patient and family.
   b. Document that informed consent was obtained.
   c. Observe the procedure, asking any questions you have.
   d. Provide post-procedure care, including:
      1. Vital signs
      2. Peripheral pulse checks
      3. Peripheral color, warmth, sensory, and motor checks
      4. Comfort measures

5. Provide care to a patient with edema. Determine the following regarding that patient:
   a. Medical diagnosis

   b. Chief complaint

   c. Cause of edema

   d. Assessment/description of edema

   e. Pertinent laboratory findings

   f. Collaborative management of edema

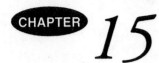

CHAPTER *15*   Nursing Management of Adults with
Arterial Disorders

1. Keep a food diary for 24 hours. Calculate your cholesterol intake. Is this intake reasonable? If it is excessive, what could you do to reduce your cholesterol intake?

2. Design three questions that could be used in collecting a nursing history to assess for the presence of arterial disorders.

3. Discuss the pathophysiology, clinical manifestations, and collaborative management for gangrene.

Continued

4. Read one journal research article related to the correlation of arterial disease and smoking. Prepare a written abstract summarizing the article.

5. Determine what programs are available in your area to assist persons to stop smoking. Compare and contrast these programs in regard to success rates, cost, and process.

6. Develop the content of a teaching plan to inform the male patient how his arterial disease could be related to his sexual dysfunction.

7. Develop the content of a teaching plan for a 78-year-old, mentally alert farmer with a third grade education who is scheduled for a PTCA.

CHAPTER

16   **Nursing Management of Adults with Hypertension**

1. Describe the characteristics of an individual with:
   a. Personality A

   b. Personality E

2. Maintain a record of your calcium and sodium intake for 48 hours. From this, estimate your daily intake of calcium (in milligrams) and your daily intake of sodium (in grams).

3. Assess your risk for developing hypertension, using the following criteria:
   a. Family history

   b. Gender

   c. Age

   d. Ethnic group

   e. Stress profile
      1. Personality characteristics

      2. Genetic factors

      3. Occupational situation

      4. Socioeconomic level

Continued

f. Dietary factors
   1. Weight

   2. Sodium

   3. Potassium

   4. Calcium

   5. Omega-3 fatty acids

g. Lifestyle habits
   1. Alcohol

   2. Smoking

   3. Physical activity

Compare the data that you have compiled with the information in the table in your text, and decide if you are at low, moderate, or high risk for developing hypertension. Decide whether any of the factors in your life are modifiable, and whether you wish to modify them. Develop a plan for modification if that is your goal.

4. Identify three patients with hypertension. Compare and contrast those persons according to:
   a. Family history of hypertension
      1.

      2.

      3.

   b. Gender
      1.

      2.

      3.

Continued

c. Age
   1.

   2.

   3.

d. Ethnic group
   1.

   2.

   3.

e. Obesity
   1.

   2.

   3.

f. Tobacco use
   1.

   2.

   3.

g. Alcohol use
   1.

   2.

   3.

h. Usual physical activity
   1.

   2.

   3.

Continued

i. Sodium intake
    1.

    2.

    3.

j. Presence of other disease
    1.

    2.

    3.

k. Occupational situation
    1.

    2.

    3.

17   **Nursing Management of Adults with
          Venous or Lymphatic Disorders**

1. List at least four nursing interventions that promote venous circulation and cite the rationale for each intervention.

2. Complete the following chart:

Name of Drug	Actions/Uses	Adverse/Side Effects and Antidote	Nursing Implications
Heparin			
Warfarin			

3. Consider the drugs heparin and coumarin as "Group A" and the drugs streptokinase, urokinase, and TPA as "Group B." Compare the two groups in regard to:
   a. Purpose/action
      1. Group A

      2. Group B

Continued

b. Risk of bleeding
   1. Group A

   2. Group B

c. Length of therapy
   1. Group A

   2. Group B

d. Side effects
   1. Group A

   2. Group B

4. Develop a teaching plan for the person on Coumadin about to be discharged home.

5. List the signs and symptoms of pulmonary embolism for which the nurse would assess in the person with DVT.

CHAPTER *18*　　**Nursing Assessment of the Cardiac System**

1. Develop a teaching plan for the person scheduled for a right-sided catheterization.

2. Explain the origin of the heart sounds.

3. Where is S_2 heard as louder? Where is S_1 heard as louder?

4. List at least three conditions that produce alterations in the heart sounds, and describe the alterations that are produced.

Condition/Disorder	Specific Alteration in Heart Sounds

Continued

5. Define *cardiac cycle* and explain the occurring events in sequence.

6. Compare and contrast stroke volume and cardiac output.

7. Perform a cardiac assessment on one person in each of the following categories: over age 80, healthy adult, adult with coronary artery disease, adult with heart valve disease. Compare and contrast your findings.

8. In the clinical setting, listen to heart sounds on five different patients for three clinical days. Discuss your findings with your peers. Ask the staff nurses to recommend patients for your study.

9. Return to the skills lab and review video/audio tapes related to heart sounds.

10. Develop a teaching plan on fats/lipids for the post-MI patient.

CHAPTER

19   **Nursing Management of Adults with Common
Complications of Cardiac Disease**

1. Nursing interventions for a patient experiencing ventricular dysrhythmia include investigating possible causes of the dysrhythmia. List five possible causes of ventricular dysrhythmia, and describe how these causes contribute to dysrhythmia.

Dysrhythmia Cause	How Cause Contribute to Dysrhythmia

2. Provide a discharge teaching plan for a patient with a permanent pacemaker.

3. You discover Mr. M. slumped in his bed. He is unresponsive when you call him and shake his shoulders. Outline the exact steps you would take in this situation in your clinical setting. Explain your rationale.

Continued

4. Answer the Critical Thinking Questions at the end of Chapter 19 in the textbook.

5. Spend a clinical day with the monitor observer. Be sure you know normal sinus rhythm and have studied Chapter 19 prior to this clinical experience. During that day, analyze a rhythm strip on each patient being monitored. Discuss your findings with the monitor observer. Be sure you understand the physiology associated with each electrical event.

6. Observe the technician performing a 12-lead ECG. In one paragraph, explain how a 12-lead ECG is used to diagnose.

7. Prioritize appropriate nursing actions for the nurse who sees a "straight line" on the patient's cardiac monitor.

8. Locate two patients with atrial fibrillation. Compare and contrast these persons in regard to:
   a. Medical diagnosis

   b. Age

   c. Cause (if known)

   d. Medications

   e. Tolerance for activity

   f. Cardiac output

Continued

9. Develop a teaching plan for a person with atrial fibrillation who is treated with anticoagulants.

10. Prioritize appropriate nursing actions for the nurse providing care to the patient whose ventricular rate suddenly drops to 32 beats per minute.

11. Prioritize appropriate nursing actions for the nurse who finds a patient in ventricular tachycardia (V-tach).

12. Prioritize appropriate nursing actions for the nurse who finds a patient in ventricular fibrillation (V-fib).

13. Compare and contrast the conditions of V-tach and V-fib.

Critical Thinking Worksheet

Name _____

 CHAPTER

20 **Nursing Management of Adults with
Disorders of the Coronary Arteries,
Myocardium, or Pericardium**

1. Plan a 24-hour menu for a post-MI patient who is on a soft, low-cholesterol, salt-restricted diet. Caffeine intake is also restricted.

2. A 58-year-old male patient who is 3 weeks post-MI tells you that he has just remarried, and verbalizes concern about sexual activity. What would you tell him?

3. A 23-year-old college student suddenly drops dead while playing volleyball, supposedly of an "enlarged heart." His coach expresses extreme guilt over the incident. "Why didn't he tell me about his heart? I could have saved him!" What could you tell this coach that might relieve some of the guilt?

4. Describe specific interventions for the management of anxiety in a patient with chest pain.

5. Develop a pre-PTCA teaching plan.

6. Draw a diagram depicting the changes in cardiac enzymes over time with an MI.

7. Develop medication cards for the following common cardiac drugs:
   a. Nitrates
   b. Beta blockers
      1. Inderal
      2. Corgard
      3. Tenormin
      4. Lopressor
   c. Calcium channel blockers
      1. Verapamil
      2. Cardizem
      3. Procardia
   d. Digoxin
   e. Anticoagulants
      1. Heparin
      2. Coumadin
      3. ASA
   f. Thrombolytics
      1. Streptokinase
      2. t-PA
   g. Lidocaine
   h. Lasix
   i. Morphine

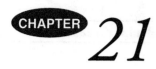 **21** **Nursing Management of Adults with Endocardial Disorders**

1. Complete the following chart:

Disorder	Defect	Pathophysiology
Mitral Stenosis		
Mitral Regurgitation		
Aortic Stenosis		
Tricuspid Stenosis		

2. Compare and contrast each of the following surgical procedures used to correct endocardial disorders:
   a. Commissural fusion

   b. Valvuloplasty

   c. Xenograft

   d. Annuloplasty

3. Provide care to one person with heart valve disease and one person with nonvalvular heart disease. Compare and contrast these persons in regard to:

	Valve disease	Nonvalvular disease
Medical diagnosis		
Symptoms		
Diagnostic studies		
Medications		

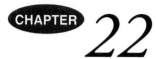

22   Nursing Assessment of the Hematologic System

1. Why is IM nonradioactive B_{12} administered to a patient who is undergoing a Schilling test?

2. Explain what is meant by a "shift to the left" in an examination of white blood cells.

3. During the collection of historical data, the nurse inquires about persistence of wounds. Why is this necessary?

4. Compare and contrast the following terms in relation to the site of origin:
   a. Hematuria

   b. Hemoptysis

   c. Hematemesis

5. Explain the effects of erythropoietin on RBC production. What would this mean for the person with renal failure? Why?

6. Explain the relationship between platelets and clotting factors. Explain how they work together and how they differ.

7. Develop a chart to carry in your pocket during clinical experiences which contains helpful information about the CBC. A suggested format is presented below.

CBC (Complete Blood Count)

Component	Lab Value	Clinical Significance
RBC		
Hg		
Hct		
Platelets		
WBC		
Neutrophils		
Bands		
Lymphocytes		
Monocytes		
Eosinophils		
Basophils		

8. Compare and contrast CBC reports of four patients, one from each of the following categories: over age 80, with active infection, with cancer, with dehydration.

9. Compare and contrast the lab tests related to bleeding disorders of two patients, one perioperative and one receiving anticoagulant therapy.

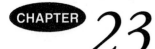 **Nursing Management of Adults with Hematologic Disorders**

1. Maintain a 24-hour record of dietary intake. On the basis of this diary, estimate your dietary intake of:
   a. Iron

   b. Vitamin K

   c. Calcium

2. Your daily intake of iron is   _____ adequate or

                                          _____ inadequate.

   Your daily intake of Vitamin K is   _____ adequate or

                                          _____ inadequate.

   Your daily intake of calcium is   _____ adequate or

                                          _____ inadequate.

3. Your patient has a disorder of the WBCs. What signs and symptoms would signal that this patient has an infection?

4. What nursing interventions could you take to prevent or control bleeding in a patient with a coagulation disorder?

Continued

5. Compare and contrast the pathophysiology, clinical manifestations, and interventions for the various anemias.

Anemia	Pathophysiology	Clinical Manifestations	Interventions
Aplastic			
Iron deficiency			
Hemolytic			
Sickle cell			
Blood loss			
Megaloblastic			
Thalassemia			

6. Compare and contrast the pathophysiology, clinical manifestations, and interventions for the various leukemias.

Leukemia	Pathophysiology	Clinical Manifestations	Interventions
AML			
ALL			
CML			
CLL			

7. Explain DIC. Include etiology, symptoms, and interventions.

8. Provide care to a person receiving blood transfusions. Assist the nurse in this procedure. Follow hospital policy and explain what you did, and the rationale, to your peers.

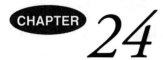

24 Nursing Assessment of the Immune System

1. Compare and contrast T Cell- and B Cell-mediated immunity in regard to:

	T Cell	B Cell
Cells involved		
Activation trigger		
Process/function		

2. Compare and contrast the nonspecific and specific immune responses.

3. Explain how corticosteroids interfere with the immune response.

4. Analyze the lab reports on three persons receiving chemotherapy. How do their WBC/diff reports differ from normal? Check for any other reports related to the immune system.

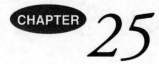

CHAPTER

25 Nursing Management of Adults with Immune Disorders

1. Explain at least five protective actions the nurse would implement for the immune-suppressed patient, and give the rationale for each.

   a.

   b.

   c.

   d.

   e.

2. Explain why persons with HIV are particularly susceptible to opportunistic infections and malignancies.

3. Provide care to a person with HIV.
   a. What self-protective measures did you take, and why?

   b. What protective measures did you implement for the patient, and why?

Continued

c. What psychosocial needs did you identify?

d. What measures did you use to address those psychosocial needs?

e. What attitudes did you observe in other health care workers toward the patient with HIV?

f. What did you teach the person with HIV?

g. What did the person with HIV teach you?

4. Develop a discharge care plan for the significant other/family of a person nearing death from HIV. Be sure to address these issues:
   a. Nutrition

   b. ADLs (bath, oral hygiene)

Continued

c. Incontinence care

d. Cleaning of eating utensils, linens, clothing, bathroom

e. Sexual activity (safe vs. unsafe)

f. Protection of care giver

5. Provide care to a person with SLE, RA, or myasthenia gravis. Assess how disease has altered his or her life in regard to:
    a. Physical mobility

    b. Physical appearance

    c. Independence

    d. Socialization

Continued

e. Pain

f. Employment

6. Describe the expected clinical manifestations and appropriate intervention measures with rationales for systemic anaphylaxis.

Clinical Manifestations	Interventions

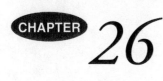

26   Nursing Assessment of the Renal and Urinary Systems

1. Develop a teaching plan for the person scheduled for renal angiography.

2. Explain the physiologic basis for the following urinalysis findings:
   a. Protein

   b. Low specific gravity

   c. Low rate of creatinine clearance

3. Compare and contrast the following symptoms:
   a. Pyuria

   b. Dysuria

   c. Oliguria

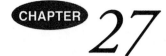

27   **Nursing Management of Adults with Renal Disorders**

1. Since dietary management is an important component in the collaborative management of patients with renal calculi, knowledge of dietary sources of calcium, phosphorus, oxalate, and purines is essential. Complete the following chart, listing foods to be avoided (high in the named substance) and foods that can be freely ingested (low in the dietary substance):

Electrolyte	Foods to Avoid	Foods That Can Be Freely Ingested
Purines		
Calcium		
Phosphorus		
Oxalates		

2. For patients with ARF and CRF, electrolyte balance is a constant concern. Knowledge of the signs and symptoms of electrolyte imbalance is essential. Complete the following chart in relation to various electrolytes:

Electrolyte	Normal Laboratory Values	Clinical Manifestations of Excess or Deficit	Nursing Management
Potassium			
Calcium			
Phosphorus			

Continued

3. A patient on hemodialysis complains of nausea and asks where he is and who you are. What interventions should you initiate at this point?

4. A patient is admitted with a diagnosis of renal colic. On admission, he is apprehensive and complains of "soreness." What assessments and interventions are appropriate at this time?

5. Observe and participate in patient care at a hemodialysis unit. Discuss the following with the nurses:
   a. Importance of predialysis body weight, BP, electrolytes, CBC

   b. Administration of blood transfusions during dialysis

   c. Incidence of potentially fatal symptoms during dialysis, and why

Continued

d. Which medications are filtered out during dialysis

e. Cumulative effect of medications during non-dialysis days

f. Psychosocial effects of hemodialysis

g. Cost of hemodialysis in terms of dollars, time, and change of lifestyle

h. Hemodialysis vs. peritoneal dialysis

I. Dialysis vs. kidney transplant

6. Develop a discharge teaching plan for the person who has renal calculi.

7. Explain the rationale for treating renal failure patients exhibiting hyperkalemia with insulin. What substance is administered with the insulin, and why? What type of insulin would you expect to be ordered, and why?

Continued

CHAPTER *28*   **Nursing Management of Adults with Urinary Tract Disorders**

1. Describe how the following factors contribute to the development of urinary tract infections:
   a. Bubble bath and perfumed soap

   b. High sugar consumption

   c. Sexual intercourse

   d. Delayed urination

2. Your patient asks for information regarding position during intercourse that will minimize pressure on the anterior vagina. What could you tell her?

3. How does acidification of the urine discourage bacterial multiplication?

4. Discuss with the gerontology clinical nurse specialist various methods of dealing with urinary incontinence in the elderly. Share this information with your classmates.

5. Communicate to the staff nurses your need to perform catheterization. Review the procedure. Practice with the skills lab models.

6. As you administer a patient's first dose of Pyridium to relieve the burning associated with UTI, what information is it important to relay to the patient?

CHAPTER *29*   **Nursing Assessment of the Neurologic System**

1. Why would a patient with right-sided hemiparesis following a stroke have profound speech difficulties?

2. Describe, specifically, how you would assess the functioning of the:
   a. Oculomotor nerves

   b. Facial nerves

   c. Olfactory nerves

3. A patient is scheduled for a lumbar puncture. The patient is alert, oriented, and very anxious. What would you say to this patient to prepare him for the procedure?

4. What questions could you ask that would check a patient's orientation to time, person, and place?

5. Perform a neuro assessment on three patients, one from each of the following categories: over age 80, para- or quadriplegia, mental disorientation. Compare and contrast your findings.

6. Develop a list of the objects needed to perform a complete neuro assessment. Write the list below, and also post it on the nursing unit where supplies are kept.

7. Accompany a patient to a neurologic diagnostic procedure. Perform appropriate teaching and assessment.

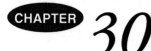

CHAPTER 30 Nursing Management of Adults with Common Neurologic Problems

1. A person begins to fall at a bus depot. You help by easing her to the ground, realizing that she is having a tonic-clonic seizure. What should you do next? What observations would it be important for you to chart?

2. List drugs that are used to treat generalized seizures and those that are used to treat partial seizures.

Drugs Used to Treat Generalized Seizures	Drugs Used to Treat Partial Seizures

3. What actions are used to test responses to pain in the unconscious patient?

4. What are the pathophysiologic mechanisms that produce headaches?

Continued

5. Get together with a group of classmates to play a game of "charades." On pieces of paper write the following terms for participants to demonstrate:
   a. Decerebration
   b. Decortication
   c. Plantar flexion
   d. Abduction
   e. Adduction
   f. Cheyne-Stokes respirations
   g. Ataxic breathing
   h. Cluster breathing
   I. Doll's eyes
   j. Any others you can think of

6. Perform a neuro assessment on a person who is alert and a person who is comatose. State the probable pathophysiology related to your findings.

7. Develop a guide to follow when assessing for increased intracranial pressure. Use your guide to assess two persons with that diagnosis.

8. Discuss intracranial herniation syndrome, differentiating between supratentorial and infratentorial herniation. Explain the urgency of this problem, etiologies, clinical manifestations, and interventions.

9. Explain how the nurse implements the order for "seizure precautions."

31   **Nursing Management of Adults with Degenerative Disorders**

1. Compare and contrast the following symptoms in Alzheimer's disease and Parkinson's disease:
   a. Agnosia

   b. Apraxia

   c. Ataxia

   d. Dyskinesia

   e. Fasciculations

   f. Orthosis

   g. Dystonia

2. Explain interventions and their rationales that are useful for patients who are prone to falling.

Continued

3. a. Which emotional state more commonly accompanies chronic disease—anxiety or depression?

    b. Describe at least three interventions that are beneficial for the patient suffering from the state in (a).

4. Alzheimer's disease was originally tagged as *premature senility*. Discuss with the gerontology clinical nurse specialist why *premature senility* is no longer an acceptable term. Explain below, and report this information back to your classmates.

5. Provide care to a patient with Alzheimer's disease. How are nursing interventions for this patient different from those for a patient with a psychiatric disorder? Why?

6. Arrange to spend clinical time in a nursing home. Compare and contrast the care of the mentally alert and the person with dementia. Also analyze the role of the nurse providing care to patients with other degenerative diseases.

7. Arrange to accompany a home health care nurse to visit a patient with Alzheimer's disease. Assess the patient and analyze the management of his or her care. Determine if further assistance is available.

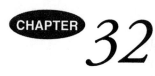

CHAPTER
32   **Nursing Management of Adults with Infectious, Inflammatory, or Autoimmune Disorders**

1. Explain why plasma exchange would be useful to a patient who has myasthenia gravis and is in crisis.

2. How would you involve the family in the care of a patient with an infectious or autoimmune disorder of the nervous system?

3. Your patient with multiple sclerosis is depressed.
   a. What clinical manifestations may indicate depression?

   b. List appropriate nursing interventions.

Continued

4. List clinical manifestations of:
    a. Bulbar weakness

    b. Meningeal irritation

    c. Cognitive impairment

5. Explain the rationale for administering Cytoxan (an anti-cancer drug) to a person with an autoimmune disease such as MS.

6. Compare and contrast multiple sclerosis and Guillain-Barré syndrome in regard to:

	MS	GBS
Etiology		
Clinical manifestations		
How diagnosed		
Interventions		
Prognosis		

7. Discuss the role of the thymus gland in regard to myasthenia gravis:
    a. As a possible contributing factor to the disease

    b. Thymectomy as an intervention

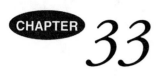

Nursing Management of Adults with Cerebrovascular Disorders

1. A number of terms are used to describe neurologic dysfunctions in the stroke victim. Define the following terms in relation to the appropriate part of the brain:
   a. Apraxia

   b. Anosognosia

   c. Dystonia

   d. Broca's aphasia

   e. Wernicke's aphasia

   f. Hemianopsia

2. Why are patients with left-sided involvement said to have a right CVA?

3. Develop a nursing care plan for a patient who has had a carotid endarterectomy.

Continued

4. Mr. Smith experienced a hemorrhagic CVA. His 30-year-old son, on discovering that Mr. Smith was not receiving heparin, said, "You people don't know what you're doing! He'll never get well without heparin to dissolve his brain clot!"

a. Identify two misconceptions under which the son is functioning.

1.

2.

b. Develop a teaching plan pertinent to this situation.

5. List and explain appropriate nursing precautions when caring for the person with a subarachnoid hemorrhage or aneurysm.

6. Visit a rehabilitation facility. Compare and contrast the care of the individual with a CVA to what you observed in the acute care setting.

 Name ____________________

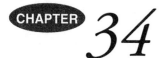

CHAPTER 34

Nursing Management of Adults with Intracranial Disorders

1. Complete the following chart regarding clinical manifestations of increased intracranial pressure:

Clinical Manifestation	Pathophysiologic Basis	Nursing Intervention
Widening pulse pressure		
Decreased pulse		
Cardiac dysrhythmias		
Headache		
Seizures		

2. Describe at least three nursing interventions that will help maintain or improve the respiratory status of a patient with a head injury.

3. A patient with a brain tumor tells you that the doctor told him he may be paralyzed after surgery. He asks you if this is true. What response could you give?

Continued

4. The father of a 14-year-old who sustained a closed head injury in a motorcycle accident says to you, "I don't trust that neurologist. He said Johnny got diabetes from the wreck. I know that's not what causes diabetes!" Develop a teaching plan related to diabetes insipidus for this family.

5. Develop a long-range care plan of appropriate guidelines for meeting the nutritional needs of a patient who is expected to remain comatose for days or even weeks. Begin with admission and plan for four weeks.

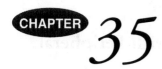

Nursing Management of Adults with Spinal Cord Disorders

1. Your patient with a spinal cord injury suddenly complains of a severe headache. Outline your nursing interventions in relation to this symptom in the order you would perform them.

2. Your young male patient has a spinal cord injury. He is depressed and says that he will not be able to have a satisfying sexual relationship with his fiancée. Develop a teaching plan related to sexual functioning for this patient and his fiancée.

3. Spend a clinical day at a rehabilitation facility. Observe and participate in teaching persons with spinal cord injuries on the following topics:
   a. ADLs
   b. Transfer techniques
   c. Bladder/bowel control techniques

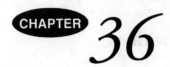

Nursing Management of Adults with Peripheral
or Cranial Nerve Disorders

1. Describe calcium disodium edetate in regard to:
   a. Classification

   b. Route of administration

   c. Side effects

   d. Interactions

   e. Nursing activities associated with drug

2. Describe how you would assess functioning of the:
   a. Trigeminal nerve

   b. Facial nerve

3. What foods would be rich in nutritional value and appropriate for a patient with facial paralysis?

4. Discuss the safety measures that need to be taught to the person with a peripheral nerve disorder affecting the lower extremities.

Name _____

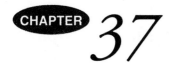

Nursing Assessment of the Eye

Following assessment of a classmate's eyes, write up your findings, using the following outline as a guide:

I. Subjective

    A. Discrepancies (if present)

        1. Specific discrepancy (use classmate's own words)

            a. Location/radiation

            b. Characteristics

            c. Sequence, duration, persistence of episode

            d. Nature of onset

            e. Associated symptoms

            f. Precipitating factors

            g. Prior episodes

    B. Examinations

    C. Medical history (past or present conditions, intervention)

    D. Family history of allergies/eye disease

    E. Medications (medication, dose, frequency)

II. Objective

    A. Visual aids

    B. External eye structures

    C. Visual acuity

    D. Color vision

    E. Visual fields

    F. Extraocular movements

    G. Pupils

    H. Appearance of cornea, iris, lens

    I. Eyegrounds (optional)

    J. Corneal light reflex

III. Nursing Diagnoses

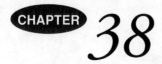

CHAPTER

38 Nursing Management of Adults with Eye Disorders

1. Describe specific ways of preventing increases in intraocular pressure after eye surgeries.

2. You have a sight-impaired patient. What specific interventions are necessary for this individual?

3. Prepare a list of general guidelines that could be used in promoting healthy vision and eyes.

Continued

4. Provide care to a patient with glaucoma. Assess the patient's knowledge related to glaucoma and reinforce appropriate self-care.

5. Perform a visual assessment on five persons over the age of 70. Compare and contrast your findings. Provide any teaching that your assessment shows is needed.

6. Arrange to accompany a home health nurse on a visit to the home of a person over age 70. Perform a visual assessment. Provide any teaching needed, make appropriate referrals, and help the person implement any safety measures needed.

7. Develop at least two plans for self-administration of medications by a visually impaired person.

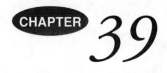

CHAPTER *39*   Nursing Assessment of the Ear

1. Compare and contrast the following terms in relation to assessment of the ear:
   a. Tinnitus

   b. Presbycusis

   c. Vertigo

   d. Cochlea

   e. Spondee

   f. Pitch

   g. Frequency

2. Explain the difference between conduction and nerve deafness.

3. How would you determine from assessment whether a patient was experiencing conduction, nerve, or mixed hearing loss?

4. Perform an auditory assessment on three persons with difficulty hearing. Compare and contrast how these persons compensate for their problem.

5. Discuss various ways nurses can be sure patients hear and understand nursing and medical instructions such as wound care and medication administration.

Nursing Management of Adults with
Ear Disorders

1. In your school or environment, spend fifteen minutes listening to sounds around you. Are these sounds that could potentially lessen hearing ability?

2. What precautions do you need to take in your professional or personal life to protect your hearing?

3. Describe care for a hearing aid.

4. Describe nursing interventions for a patient who is experiencing vertigo.

5. Inquire at your clinical facility whether a sign-language competent resource person is available for patients/families with that need.

6. Provide care to a person with difficulty hearing. What methods of communication, other than speech, did you use? Which methods were effective?

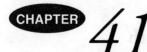

CHAPTER 41   Nursing Assessment of the
Musculoskeletal System

1. Determine which diagnostic and laboratory tests would be useful in the diagnosis of systemic lupus ery-
   thematosus, and describe them.

2. What types of movement would you expect from each of the following joints? What range-of-motion
   exercises would benefit these joints?
   a. Knee

   b. Shoulder

   c. Hip

3. What would you expect to find during physical assessment of an inflamed joint?

Continued

4. Perform a musculoskeletal assessment of five persons over age 70. Compare and contrast your findings.
   a. What nursing diagnoses did you identify?

   b. What manifestations did you assess?

   c. What compensatory measures had the persons implemented?

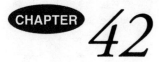

CHAPTER *42*   **Nursing Management of Adults with Musculoskeletal Trauma**

1. Many terms are used to describe fractures. Draw the fracture that is indicated by each of the following:
   a. Distal femur

   b. Depressed skull fracture

   c. Closed midshaft transverse fracture of the radius

   d. Compression fracture of the L2 vertebra

   e. Oblique intracapsular fracture of the femur

2. Describe the postoperative nursing care for a patient who has undergone closed intramedullary nailing.

Continued

3. What measures could you take to control bleeding in a patient with a below-the-knee traumatic amputation?

4. Compare and contrast sprain and strain in relation to definition, clinical manifestations, and collaborative management.

5. Identify and describe the stages of bone healing.

6. Provide care to the patient in skin traction. Discuss how you assisted the patient with the following needs:
   a. Personal hygiene

   b. Prevention of skin breakdown

   c. Nutrition

   d. Elimination

   e. Mobility

   f. Psychosocial needs

7. Provide care to the patient with an external fixation device. Narratively chart your assessment of the area involved as well as your nursing actions.

8. Compare and contrast factors to be assessed in the patient who has a cast in relation to the rationale for each factor and the appropriate nursing action for each factor.

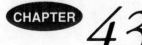

43 Nursing Management of Adults with Degenerative, Inflammatory, or Autoimmune Musculoskeletal Disorders

1. Compare and contrast clinical manifestations and interventions for the various forms of arthritis:

Type	Clinical Manifestations	Interventions
Osteoarthritis		
Rheumatoid Arthritis		
Gout		

2. Develop a discharge teaching plan for the person with rheumatoid arthritis. Be sure to include:
   a. Pain control

   b. Safety

   c. ADLs

   d. Diet

   e. Mobility

3. Develop a nutrition teaching plan for the person recently diagnosed with gout.

Continued

4. Provide care to a patient who had a hip or knee joint replaced.
   a. List the nursing diagnoses you identified.

   b. Plot out on a calendar from the pre-op period to discharge:
      1. Pain (scale of 1-10) and pain control
      2. Mobility
      3. Laboratory values

5. Compare and contrast osteoporosis and Paget's disease in regard to:

	Osteoporosis	Paget's Disease
Etiology		
Pathophysiology		
Clinical manifestations		
Interventions		

6. As a nurse you might be asked to speak to a women's group on topics of women's health. Develop a 15-minute presentation on osteoporosis, focusing on prevention. Outline your presentation here.

Continued

7. Provide care to a person who recently had bone surgery or a complicated bone fracture.
   a. What assessment criteria did you use to look for osteomyelitis?

   b. What nursing measures did you implement to prevent osteomyelitis?

   c. If the patient were to have an external fixation device, what nursing actions would you implement to prevent osteomyelitis?

8. Discuss the following patient scenario in a small group of your classmates:
   Mrs. J. was admitted with low back pain. All diagnostic test results, e.g., CT, rheumatoid factor, were negative/normal. Mrs. J. requires Demerol q4h and cries a lot. She also told you she is currently going through a divorce.
   a. How can you, as the nurse, approach the issue of pain with the physician? With the patient?

   b. Is it possible that Mrs. J. has physical pain?

44 Nursing Assessment of the Endocrine System

1. Explain the concept of negative feedback.

2. During assessment of the endocrine system, it is essential to locate the gland accurately. Draw a picture of the neck, indicating the location of the thyroid gland in relation to key anatomic landmarks.

3. List all diagnostic tests which are considered useful in the diagnosis of thyroid disorders, along with their normal values and clinical significance.

Test	Normal Value	Clinical Significance

Continued

4. Write narratively how you would chart that you were unable to palpate the thyroid in a very overweight patient.

5. You are in the process of admitting Mr. B., a person with Type I IDDM. Write narratively how you would chart that he said he takes a little insulin when he feels as if his blood sugar is up, his right big toe is swollen and draining yellow pus, he has body odor, he has an open pack of cigarettes in his shirt pocket, and his capillary blood sugar you just checked was 423.

Critical Thinking Worksheet

Name _____

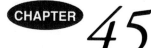

CHAPTER *45* **Nursing Management of Adults with Hypothalamus, Pituitary, or Adrenal Disorders**

1. Differentiate between diabetes mellitus and diabetes insipidus:

	DM	DI
Pathophysiology		
Clinical manifestations		
Interventions		

2. Differentiate between Addison's disease and Cushing's syndrome:

	AD	CS
Pathophysiology		
Clinical manifestations		
Interventions		

Continued

3. Develop a nursing care plan for the patient having a transphenoidal pituitary tumor resection. Include preoperative teaching and postoperative care.

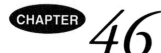

CHAPTER

46　　Nursing Management of Adults with Thyroid or
Parathyroid Disorders

1. Compare and contrast myxedema coma and thyroid storm.

2. Describe the signs and symptoms of tetany and nursing activities related to the assessment of tetany in your patient.

3. Develop three questions that could be asked during collection of a patient history to provide information about the patient's risk for thyroid disorders and/or information about functioning of the thyroid.

Continued

4. Complete the following related to Graves' disease:
   a. Also known as

   b. Etiology

   c. Pathophysiology

   d. Clinical manifestations

   e. Interventions

5. Complete the following related to hypothyroidism:
   a. Also known as

   b. Etiology

   c. Pathophysiology

   d. Clinical manifestations

   e. Interventions

6. On the evening prior to parathyroidectomy, Mrs. C.'s surgeon ordered "tracheostomy tray at bedside." How would you explain this to the patient so as to prevent alarm?

Continued

CHAPTER

47   **Nursing Management of Adults with Diabetes Mellitus**

1. Determine your caloric requirements for a day. Using this requirement as a guide, design a diabetic regimen for yourself using the exchange lists and take into account any factors that affect your eating habits and diet.

2. You are explaining possible complications to a diabetic patient. How would you explain each of the following? (Include physiologic basis and preventive measures in your explanations and use language that the patient might understand.)
   a. Risk for infection

   b. Retinopathy

   c. Coronary artery disease

3. Your newly diagnosed IDDM patient is an avid jogger and jogs 2 to 3 miles per day. How might this patient manage this aspect of her lifestyle in relation to her diabetes?

4. Compare and contrast insulin and oral hypoglycemics.

Continued

5. While providing care to your patient in a semiprivate room, you overhear the nurse tell the other patient, who is newly diagnosed with IDDM, that the insulin injections will burn the sugar he eats.
   a. What information does that nurse not possess?

   b. How might that statement influence the patient's decision regarding taking insulin when he is ill?

   c. How would you go about teaching your peer?

6. Which is the emergency of higher priority, a blood sugar of 540 or a blood sugar of 32? Why? What is the intervention?

7. Mr. Sweet's fasting blood tests revealed a serum potassium of 3.2 and a glucose of 178. Explain why the nurse contacted the physician prior to administering the insulin, since the sugar is elevated and the patient will be eating breakfast.

8. Find the policy at your clinical agency for nursing measures to treat hypoglycemic reactions. On a piece of paper, simplify the policy/procedure into sequential steps. Be sure to include specific data, e.g., how many ml of orange juice. Attach a copy to the beverage refrigerator on the unit and keep a copy for yourself.

9. Develop a teaching plan for your patient with NIDDM who says, "I give my wife one of my insulin pills when we have dessert, because she doesn't want to get fat."

10. Identify nursing strategies for managing the adolescent with IDDM who is noncompliant to his insulin and diet regimen.

CHAPTER *48*   Nursing Assessment of the
                     Gastrointestinal System

1. Consider the functions of the liver, and using this as basis, explain why it is essential to consider tests such as the platelet count and bleeding and clotting times before performing a liver biopsy.

2. A patient is having difficulty absorbing fat-soluble vitamins. This patient is scheduled for percutaneous transhepatic cholangiogram. Is this patient especially at risk for bleeding following the examination? Why or why not?

3. You suspect that psychogenic factors may be influencing a patient's abdominal pain. Design at least two questions that could elicit data that would clarify this relationship.

4. Follow starch through its digestion in the gastrointestinal system.

5. Review the lab reports of three patients with liver disease. Compare and contrast your findings. Assess the patients for manifestations related to the abnormal findings:
   a. Abnormal findings

   b. Clinical manifestations

CHAPTER *49*   **Nursing Management of Adults with Disorders of the Mouth or Esophagus**

1.   a. Compare and contrast the nursing interventions for the following surgical procedures. Include the rationale for each intervention.

.   b. Where are the following symptoms manifested?

     1. Melena

     2. Pyrosis

     3. Dysphagia

     4. Fundoplication

     5. Glossectomy

     6. Bougie

     7. Esophagogastrostomy

     8. Heller procedure

Continued

2. Eating is a common component of socialization. What emotional and social responses would you anticipate in a patient who experiences alterations in the normal patterns of eating? What interventions would
be effective with this patient? Name at least three.

3. List nursing considerations specific to the process of eating in elderly patients, including rationales.

4. Your patient's oral infection was diagnosed by the physician as "thrush." The patient is receiving an
antibiotic as a postop prophylactic measure. After the physician leaves the room, the patient asks you
why the doctor did not order another antibiotic for his mouth infection. How will you respond?

CHAPTER *50*   Nursing Management of Adults with
Disorders of the Stomach or Duodenum

1. Outline all the clinical manifestations of bleeding in a patient with bleeding from the stomach or duodenum.

2. Outline the clinical manifestations of perforation. Describe what you would do if your patient with a gastric ulcer showed signs of perforation.

3. Why is vitamin B_{12} deficiency a concern after gastric surgeries?

4. Determine special precautions in administering cimetidine and ranitidine to elderly patients. Describe these precautions.

Continued

5. Return to the skills lab and practice inserting nasogastric tubes. Review from your fundamentals text the following:
   a. Gavage
   b. Lavage
   c. Salem-sump
   d. Levine tube
   e. Continuous vs. intermittent gastric suction
   f. Miller-Abbott tube
   g. Sengstaken-Blakemore tube

6. Review the various parenteral feeding products, e.g., Jevity, Sustacal. If your patient develops diarrhea, what will you do?

7. List the expected clinical manifestations of peritonitis. State in one brief paragraph the significance of peritonitis and its treatment.

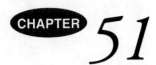

CHAPTER 51   **Nursing Management of Adults with Intestinal Disorders**

1. Explain the physiologic basis for complications arising from an abdominal resection with permanent colostomy.

Complication	Physiologic Basis
Urinary retention	
Pelvic abscess	
Sexual dysfunction	

2. Describe three deviations in the normal appearance of a stoma, and describe nursing activities in relation to these deviations.

Deviation	Nursing Activities

Continued

3. What type of drainage is expected from a(n):
   a. Ileostomy

   b. Descending colostomy

   c. Transverse loop colostomy

4. A patient experiences an altered body image following colostomy. The patient refuses to look at the stoma or perform self-care. Develop a care plan that helps this patient deal with his altered self-image.

Continued

5. Provide care to a patient with a bowel diversion or colostomy.
   a. When assessing the stoma, what factors did you observe?

   b. How did you maintain nutrition for the patient?

   c. Describe stoma care you provided.

   d. Discuss the patient's psychosocial response to the diversion.

   e. Discuss the teaching needed by the patient.

   f. What did you learn from the enterostomal therapist?

6. Explain why, from a pathophysiologic perspective, an intestinal obstruction is so significant.

7. The surgeon removes the abdominal dressing from the patient who had a descending colostomy yester-day, and you observe two stomas approximately 4 inches apart.
   a. Explain what each stoma is.

   b. Explain how the replacement sterile dressing should be applied.

8. Spend a day with the enterostomal therapist. Be sure to accomplish the following:
   a. Observe how to maintain psychosocial dignity for the patient.
   b. Observe the therapist change an ostomy pouch.
   c. Observe the therapist teaching the patient.

Critical Thinking Worksheet

Name _____

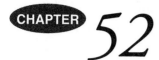

CHAPTER 52

Nursing Management of Adults with Disorders of the Liver, Biliary Tract, or Exocrine Pancreas

1. Complete the following chart:

Clinical Manifestation of Cirrhosis	Physiologic Basis for Clinical Manifestation
Ascites	
Bleeding	
Jaundice	
Anemia	
Esophageal varices	

2. Why would vitamin K be necessary for a patient who will be undergoing a cholecystectomy?

3. Develop three questions that could be used in a nursing history and would be useful in differentiating the clinical manifestations of pancreatitis from those of cholecystitis.

4. Explain why the patient with cirrhosis, who already has a low serum albumin level, is placed on a low protein or no protein diet.

5. Explain why the nurse would not omit a dose of Lactulose for the patient with cirrhosis whose ammonia level is elevated, even though he has developed diarrhea.

6. Discuss with the infection control nurse the risk of hepatitis in nurses. Be sure to discuss prevention and consequences. Share this information with your classmates.

7. Discuss the ethical and financial considerations of liver transplant for the person with cirrhosis related to alcohol abuse. What about the person with massive damage from hepatitis?

8. Provide care for the person having a cholecystectomy.
   a. Compare and contrast the course of therapy by traditional surgery vs. laser surgery.

   b. Explain the function of the T-tube.

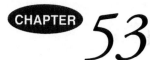

53 Nursing Assessment of the Reproductive System

1. Outline the changes that occur in the female reproductive tract as a result of aging.

2. Outline the changes that occur in the male reproductive tract as a result of aging.

3. Define the following terms in relation to the male or female reproductive system:
   a. Cremasteric reflex

   b. FSH

   c. Areolae

   d. ELISA

   e. RPR

4. On a sheet of paper, develop a calendar for one month and plot out the phases and events of the uterine cycle.

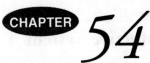

CHAPTER

54   Sexuality and Reproductive Health

1. You are to collect a sexual history from a 30-year-old woman. List at least six questions that you could use and then discuss how you would conduct the interview in such a way as to facilitate the comfort of the patient.

2. Define the following terms:
   a. Tumescence

   b. Contraception

   c. Dyspareunia

3. Ask the nurses at your clinical facility if pap smear and BSE teaching services are available for female patients who desire them. If it is available and if your patient's doctor approves, offer these services to your patient.

4. Admit four patients, two males (one elderly) and two females (one elderly). Obtain a sexual history and assessment of each within the admitting process.

5. Discuss possible nursing actions which would accommodate normal sexual function of persons in the nursing home environment.

6. Develop a teaching plan for the male who complains of impotence.

7. Discuss with the physician the normal sexual needs of your patient who is experiencing prolonged hospitalization. With the physician's permission, make arrangements for privacy during spousal visits. Discuss with your peers whether this accommodation should be made available to the patient who is homosexual.

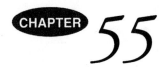

CHAPTER *55*   **Nursing Management of Women with Reproductive System Disorders**

1. Describe the procedure for BSE.

2. Postmenopausal women experience dyspareunia as a result of changes in the vagina. Discuss these changes and what you could suggest that would make intercourse less painful.

3. Describe the rationale for maintaining a patient who is receiving internal irradiation on bed rest and in low-Fowler's position.

Continued

4. Explain why women with PID are sometimes treated in an uncaring, degrading manner.

5. List the clinical manifestations of PMS and the pathophysiologic causes thought to exist.

6. Prepare an explanation for the patient with uterine cancer who says, "I can't possibly have cancer there—my pap smear last month was normal!"

7. Describe the "typical" breast cancer patient.

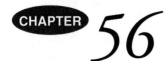

CHAPTER 56 **Nursing Management of Men with Reproductive System Disorders**

1. Explain the term "retrograde ejaculation."

2. Explain why inhibition of androgen synthesis in the testes and adrenals or blockage of androgenic responses in the prostate might slow or reverse cancer of the prostate.

3. Describe nursing interventions that will assist healing of the anastomosis in a radical prostatectomy; give the rationale for each intervention.

4. Describe how you would explain testicular self-examination to a patient.

5. Develop a teaching plan for the patient having a transurethral resection of the prostate (TURP). Include the following factors:

a. 3-way catheter

b. Forcing fluids

c. Long-term sexual consequences

6. Develop a teaching plan for the patient with prostatic cancer who will be receiving estrogen therapy.

CHAPTER 57
Nursing Management of Adults with Sexually Transmitted Diseases

1. What STDs are reportable in your state/county/province?

2. How do you report STDs?

3. What, if any, support groups or organizations exist in your community for patients with AIDS? What services do these groups provide? How might patients contact these groups or organizations?

4. What response would you give to a patient with an STD who says, "I am no good. Look at the harm I've caused my wife. I'll never be able to face her or my family again"?

Continued

5. Compare and contrast the following STDs:

STD	Etiology	Clinical Manifestations	Treatments
Chlamydia			
Herpes genitalis			
Gonorrhea			
Syphilis			
Chancroid			
Genital warts			
Trichomoniasis			
Vaginal candidiasis			

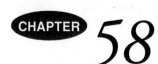

CHAPTER *58*   Nursing Assessment of the
Integumentary System

1. Use each of the following terms correctly in a sentence that would appear in charting related to assessment of the integument:
   a. Ecchymosis

   b. Keloids

   c. Lentigines

   d. Pruritus

   e. Striae

2. In the intradermal skin test, what would signify hypersensitivity to the injected allergen?

3. List at least five findings during assessment of the integument that could be related to conditions other than skin disorders.

4. List skin assessment techniques and characteristics specific to:
   a. Persons with dark skin

   b. The elderly

5. Perform a skin assessment on five patients, each meeting one of the following criteria: dark skin, white skin, elderly, with a decubitus, with a surgical wound. Compare and contrast your findings.

6. Go to the hospital or school of nursing library and obtain a book with photographs of skin disorders. Select ten different photos and narratively chart a description of each as if they appeared on patients in your care.

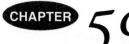

CHAPTER *59*   **Nursing Management of Adults with Skin Disorders**

1. Outline precautions that can be taken to lessen sun exposure or damage from sun exposure.

2. Outline how you would prepare a:
   a. Cornstarch bath

   b. Soda bicarbonate bath

   c. Potassium permanganate bath

3. Mrs. M. is 80 years old and has Alzheimer's disease. She spends hours sitting in a chair in the hallway and must be toileted by nursing staff. What is her risk for development of pressure sores?

4. Retin-A is a current remedy for the treatment of aging skin. Outline its action, uses, side effects, and application.

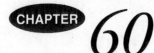

Nursing Management of Adults with Burns

1. A patient has experienced burns to the face, neck, anterior trunk, and both arms and hands. Estimate the extent of burn injury, using the:
   a. Rule of nines

   b. Lund and Browder chart

2. Describe how fingers and hands that have been burned should be wrapped, and why.

3. Explain why 5% dextrose is used in the resuscitation of the adult burn patient.

4. Explain why partial-thickness burns are more painful than full-thickness burns.

Continued

5. Explain which collaborative measures are taken to promote burn wound healing and the rationale for each.

Collaborative Treatment	Rationale

6. Describe the body's response to severe burns (and give the rationale for each) in regard to:

	Response	Rationale
Cardiovascular		
Pulmonary		
Renal		
Gastrointestinal		
Hematopoietic		

Continued

	Response	Rationale
Neurologic		
Endocrine		
Metabolic		

7. Discuss the added complexity of the burn victim having pre-existing IDDM, CHF, or emphysema.

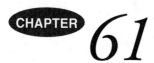

Nursing Management of Adults Undergoing Cosmetic or Reconstructive Surgery

1. Define the following terms:
   a. Blepharoplasty

   b. Decubitus ulcer

   c. Pedicle flap

   d. Rhytidectomy

   e. Blow-out fracture

2. Describe nursing treatments that are useful in caring for a patient who has a poor body image.

3. Prepare a list of liquids that would be appropriate for a patient with jaw wiring.

Continued

4. List specific nursing measures, with rationales, to ensure airway patency for the patient who has undergone mandibular wiring.

5. Discuss third-party payment for cosmetic and reconstructive surgery with a representative from a large insurance company. What did you learn?

Case Studies

The Patient with Chronic Obstructive Pulmonary Disease, Having an Episode of Acute Respiratory Distress

Mrs. Antonio, a 69-year-old woman with a long history of chronic obstructive pulmonary disease, is having an episode of acute respiratory distress. Upon admission to the hospital, Mrs. Antonio's breathing is labored, with rapid shallow respirations and use of accessory muscles to breathe. She has an anxious and exhausted look in her eyes. Her skin is dusky. She is 5' 6" and weighs 102 pounds. She is known to the nursing staff, having been hospitalized once or twice a year with similar symptoms.

1. What will the nurse include in the admission assessment of Mrs. Antonio?

After chest x-rays and arterial blood gases are done, Mrs. Antonio is diagnosed as having acute respiratory failure with pneumothorax. Her physician inserts a chest tube and an endotracheal tube and begins mechanical ventilation.

2. What data (subjective, objective, and laboratory) should be used by the nurse to evaluate this patient's response to this therapy?

Mrs. Antonio's physician orders drug and nutritional therapy: intravenous aminophylline, inhaled beta agonists, intravenous corticosteroids, low dose subcutaneous heparin, stress ulcer prophylaxis, formulated gavage tube feedings and crystalloid intravenous fluids.

Continued

3. Given Mrs. Antonio's presenting condition, what should the nurse understand about the rationale for each of these therapies?

4. What will the nurse include in this patient's assessment as long as she is being mechanically ventilated?

5. What will the nurse include in this patient's assessment while she is receiving formulated gavage tube feedings?

After 3 weeks, Mrs. Antonio's condition has improved, and she is recuperating satisfactorily.

6. What key points should the nurse review with Mrs. Antonio to help her limit future exacerbations of her pulmonary disease?

Name _____

The Patient with Tuberculosis

Richard is a 28-year-old male who has come to the hospital with complaints of fever, cough, night sweats, malaise, weight loss, anorexia and fatigue. Social and medical history: he was a teenage runaway and lived as a street person for 5 years; he sometimes uses illegal drugs. Six years ago he married and took a minimum wage job working in a textile factory where many immigrants from third world countries are employed. Three years ago he was diagnosed and treated for pulmonary tuberculosis. Richard, his wife, and three children share a three-bedroom home with another family of five.

1. Identify the risk factors associated with tuberculosis that this patient has experienced.

In order to diagnose Richard, the physician orders chest x-ray studies, pulmonary function tests and sputum microscopic examinations and cultures.

2. What should the nurse know about these diagnostic tools and their limitations with patients suspected of having or having tuberculosis?

3. What key factors should the nurse evaluate about Richard when considering his discharge planning?

Name _____

The Patient with Primary Hypertension

Mr. George is a 50-year-old male who has recently retired. He was diagnosed as having primary hypertension 3 years ago. Although he has been seeing a doctor, his blood pressure has continued to rise. Recently the company physician insisted on an early retirement. Mr. George is a classic personality E. His friends nicknamed him "Archie Bunker." He is 5' 10" and weighs 209 pounds. He brags about being a "six pack-a-day man."

1. Do a risk assessment for hypertension on Mr. George.

Mr. George talks about his prescribed medical regimen in very contemptuous tones. Occasionally his concern for his health manifests itself in questions about the effects of high blood pressure.

2. List six of the complications that Mr. George could develop if his hypertension goes untreated.

3. Identify some strategies the nurse could use to enhance Mr. George's compliance with suggested lifestyle modifications.

The Patient with Parkinson's Disease

Mrs. Norris is a 76-year-old woman who has been admitted to the hospital because her physician has decided to place her on a "drug holiday." Mrs. Norris was first diagnosed 22 years ago as having Parkinson's disease. She has had progressive loss of postural reflexes and has suffered several falls. She prefers to spend most of her day in bed. To leave home she uses a wheelchair. She has a live-in helper 5 days a week.

1.   What should the nurse include in this patient's admission assessment?

Mrs. Norris was living alone at home when she was diagnosed as having Parkinson's. Her only family is a daughter who lives and works in a city 80 miles away. The daughter comes home on weekends to care for Mrs. Norris. The daughter reveals her concerns about how much longer it will be practical and safe to let her mother remain at home.

2.   What considerations should the nurse help the daughter identify in making this decision?

3.   What special care is Mrs. Norris likely to need while she is weaned from her dopaminergic drugs?

The Patient with a Cerebrovascular Accident

Mrs. King, 85 years old, has been admitted to the hospital with a diagnosis of suspected cerebrovascular accident. She lives in her own home with her husband, who is a year older. The couple had been able to meet their own daily needs with minimal help from grown children who visit regularly.

1. What elements of the admission assessment are important for this client?

Diagnostic examinations confirm what the physician calls a small ischemic CVA affecting limited areas of the right hemisphere and a high occlusion of the middle cerebral artery.

2. What dysfunctions are typical of right hemisphere CVA?

The physician tells Mr. King and the family that they should consider admitting Mrs. King to a long-term facility. Mr. King rejects this idea and insists that he wants to try caring for his wife in their home.

Continued

3. What resources could the nurse suggest to help him with this undertaking?

Mrs. King has no motor function deficits, but she has homonymous hemianopsia.

4. What safety hazard could this present?

Name _____

The Patient with Lumbar Intervertebral Disk Disease

Mark is a 34-year-old male with a herniated nucleus pulposus of L4 to L5. He was very active as a youth, playing football in high school. While in the Marine Corps he trained with a special forces unit. After military service he tried a number of jobs that involved heavy weight lifting. Four years ago he decided to become a nurse. He has 6 weeks of nursing school left to finish. Last weekend he was struck with sharp low back pain while cranking his lawn mower. Mark describes his pain as starting in his lower back and running down his buttock to his left thigh.

1. What additional data should the nurse obtain?

Mark's physician agrees to allow him to return to school and "light duty" after only 1 week of bed rest. He is given prescriptions for analgesics, muscle relaxants and anti-inflammatory agents.

2. What information should be stressed to Mark for safe self-administration of these medications while he is attending school?

3. What nonpharmacologic measures could the nurse suggest to Mark to help with his condition?

Name _____

The Patient with Right Above-Knee Amputation

C.C., a 67-year-old single, retired real estate agent, has a long history of cardiovascular disease due to generalized atherosclerosis. He also has hypertension and COPD (with home oxygen). He has been receiving home health services since he was discharged from the hospital after an axillary-bifemoral graft for peripheral vascular occlusion in both legs. During this hospital stay, the patient required a transmetatarsal amputation of the left foot. The patient complained to the home health nurse that he had an acute onset of right calf pain with numbness, pain, loss of movement, and coldness of the right lower leg and foot. The home health nurse notified the physician, who ordered Mr. C.C. to go to the local hospital for a vascular scan. The scan showed complete occlusion of the right side of the axillary-bifemoral graft, and he was admitted to SICU in preparation for a right above-knee amputation. After an uneventful surgery, Mr. C.C. returned home 2 weeks later with a bandaged stump.

The physician ordered skilled nursing visits daily for 4 weeks for dressing changes and venipuncture; then three times a week for 4 weeks; PT three times a week for 8 weeks; and home health aides three times a week for 8 weeks.

1. What should the nurse include in the initial assessment regarding safety issues?

2. Describe the technique of preparing the amputation site for a prosthesis.

3. What type of body image changes would Mr. C.C. experience? Develop nursing diagnoses that would direct your plan of care.

The Patient with a Total Hip Replacement

Mr. Petry, a 72-year-old man, was admitted for a total hip replacement. He had a total hip replacement 4 years ago. Two years ago he fell on the affected hip and subsequently developed an infection. Eighteen months ago he had an endoprosthesis removal. Treatment of the infection is finally successful. He is scheduled to get another total hip replacement tomorrow.

1. What should be included in his preoperative instruction?

2. What assessments should be made by the nurse while monitoring Mr. Petry's postoperative recovery?

Continued

3. What does the nurse assess regarding dislocation?

4. What should the nurse do if excessive blood loss is suspected?

Name _____

The Patient with Osteoarthritis

M.T., a 70-year-old widow, was being serviced by the local home health agency for activity intolerance related to osteoarthritis. During a skilled-nurse visit, the nurse found Mrs. M.T. to have 3+ to 4+pedal edema in the left leg. Pedal pulses were present in both extremities. The patient was complaining of severe pain in the left knee. The physician ordered Mrs. M.T. to come to the office for an injection of cortisone.

1. Develop a teaching plan to focus on care of the knee after the cortisone.

2. What measures can be taken to reduce further exacerbations of knee pain?

3. What safety measures must be instituted for the patient who has osteoarthritis?

The Patient with Hypothyroidism

Mrs. Quinones is an 80-year-old woman with Hashimoto's thyroiditis. The disease was diagnosed when she was in her middle 40s. When her family doctor died 25 years ago, Mrs. Quinones continued hormone replacement with medication she purchased twice a year in a Mexican border town 150 miles from her home. Six months ago Mrs. Quinones began seeing a cardiologist. Her complaints were headache, activity intolerance, dependent edema and shortness of breath. The physician diagnosed hypertension, congestive heart failure, and chronic atrial fibrillation.

1. What is the probable connection between Mrs. Quinones' thyroid condition and her more recent cardio-vascular problems?

Mrs. Quinones has been admitted to the coronary care unit after several fainting episodes. When she initially came to the emergency room, her skin was cold, clammy, and dusky colored, and she had pulmonary congestion. It was found that she had paroxysmal atrial tachycardia.

2. What risk factors make Mrs. Quinones a candidate for the complication of myxedema coma, even with prompt treatment of her cardiac problem?

Continued

3. Mrs. Quinones could be expected to have several changes indicative of inadequate thyroid hormone replacement. Identify classic signs of hypothyroidism.

4. What information should the nurse be sure Mrs. Quinones has in order to self-administer her thyroid supplement when she goes home?

Name _____

The Patient with Insulin-dependent Diabetes Mellitus

You are working in an outpatient ambulatory ED center when a mother brings in her 20-year old daughter, C.J., who has type I diabetes mellitus and has just returned from a trip to Mexico. She's had a 3-day FUO (fever of unknown origin), and diarrhea with nausea and vomiting. She has been unable to eat and has tolerated only sips of fluid. Because she has been unable to eat, she has not taken her insulin.

Because C.J. is unsteady, you bring her to the examining room in a wheelchair. While assisting her onto the examining table, you note that her skin is very warm and flushed. Her respirations are deep and rapid, and her breath is foul smelling. C.J. is drowsy and unable to answer your questions. Her mother states, "She keeps telling me she's so thirsty, but she can't keep anything down."

1.   Describe the pathophysiology of diabetic ketoacidosis.

The nurse checked C.J.'s blood sugar with a glucometer. The reading was 347 mg/dl. The physician ordered 1000 mg LR IV stat, 35 units of Lente and 20 units of regular insulin SC now. He also placed her on a sliding scale. He ordered that C.J. be transported to the local hospital.

2.   What is the rationale behind using an infusion pump for the IV solution?

C.J. is ready for transport to the medical ICU. Her mother is beginning to realize that C.J. is more severely ill than she thought. She leaves the room and begins to cry.

3.   How would you handle this situation?

4.   The mother asks where she can get more information on how C.J. can control her diabetes. What are some resources she may find useful?

Name _____

The Patient with Decubitus Ulcer

O.G. is an 89-year-old bedridden patient receiving home health services for multiple system problems. She had a CVA 5 years ago that left her with speech and mobility deficits on the left side. She has severe contractures that leave her in a fetal position. She has a PEG tube for tube feeding, a urinary catheter, and TED stockings. Because of her bedridden condition, she has developed decubiti on both hips at the head of the trochanter. Both decubiti are approximately 2 to 3 inches in circumference and 1½ inches in depth.

1. How do you assess the wounds for healing process?

2. Describe the wound care procedure for this type of wound.

3. What measures are done to promote adequate circulation to prevent further development of pressure sores?

Name _____

The Patient with Liver Failure

Mr. Trisch is a 48-year-old lawyer. He is married and has an 18-year-old daughter. Early today he vomited a large amount of blood and fainted in his home. He was brought to the hospital by ambulance. His wife and daughter accompanied him. Mr. Trisch's physician diagnosed a hemorrhage of esophageal varices secondary to Laennec's cirrhosis. Balloon tamponade is used to control the bleeding.

1. Discuss the role of the nurse in caring for a patient with a Sengstaken-Blakemore tube.

Mr. Trisch's condition stabilizes, and 12 hours after his admission he is taken for endoscopic injection sclerotherapy. The procedure is tolerated well and Mr. Trisch's esophageal bleeding is controlled.

2. What complications could have occurred in the period between his admission and the successful sclerotherapy?

Continued

3. What measures should the nurse anticipate would be ordered to prevent or control these complications?

Mr. Trisch's condition continues to improve and he talks enthusiastically with his wife about adopting a healthier lifestyle. The nurse overhears him say, "I can't wait to eat all the steaks I can sink my teeth into!"

4. What should the nurse clarify about his daily protein intake?

5. What measures could the nurse take to help Mrs. Trisch and her daughter learn about their roles in Mr. Trisch's alcohol problem as well as his recovery?

The Patient with Prostate Cancer

C.P. is a 68-year-old married farmer with a past medical history of smoking for 40 years. He was admitted to the hospital for progressive cough and chest congestion. Despite a week of antibiotic therapy, C.P. continued to worsen; he experienced progressive dyspnea and productive cough, and began to have night sweats. He also told the physician that he has a history of lower back pain and decreased ability to urinate. The physician ordered a chest x-ray and a PSA. The chest x-ray revealed a left hilar lung mass, probable lung cancer. The PSA was grossly elevated. The physician diagnosed prostatic cancer with metastasis to C.P.'s lungs. After the physician discussed the prognosis with both C.P. and his family members, C.P. decided that he did not want to go have chemotherapy or radiation therapy. The physician then referred him to hospice care.

1. Develop a teaching plan to focus on pain management for C.P.

2. During the initial assessment, the nurse discovered that C.P. is a devout Catholic. What measures will be taken to ensure that C.P.'s spiritual needs will be met?

C.P. began to experience an elevated temperature of 101 degrees accompanied by decreased breath sounds in all lobes. His breathing became more labored with periods of apnea. The family members called the hospice nurse.

3. What actions did the hospice nurse take at this time?

The Patient with Prostate Cancer

Critical
Thinking
Guides

The application of critical thinking is promoted in the algorithms or critical thinking guides provided in this section. By applying critical thinking to these specific patient situations, the student will be encouraged to develop decision-making skills in the clinical environment. These guides lead the student visually and mentally through pathways of patient care, showing the student the process the nurse follows in gathering, organizing, and evaluating patient data. The student can then plan nursing interventions and patient teaching to improve skill as a nurse and foster better patient outcomes.

Critical Thinking Guide

The Patient with Essential Hypertension

Look at the accompanying critical thinking guide and provide the appropriate information for the shaded boxes.

Mr. James Rockwell is a 54-year-old black male who has recently complained of dizziness. He visited his physician, who was concerned about a blood pressure reading of 170/110 on his first visit. Mr. Rockwell returned the following day to have his blood pressure retested by the nurse. At that time his blood pressure was 160/106. He scheduled a follow-up visit with his physician the following week. At that time his blood pressure was 182/118.

Mr. Rockwell is very concerned about his blood pressure. His grandfather, father, and brothers have had high blood pressure and are treated with medication. His grandfather recently had a stroke. Mr. Rockwell has meant to have his blood pressure tested for several years, but could never seem to find the time. His wife complains that he is a workaholic. He is under a great deal of stress both at work and at home. He does not pay much attention to his diet, as he has little time for healthy meals or exercise. His diet consists mostly of fast foods and coffee. He knows this has to change because he is approximately 25 pounds overweight, especially in the abdominal area. Like many men of his generation, he smokes 2 packs of cigarettes per day. He would like to quit, but smoking helps him deal with the daily stress he experiences.

Mr. Rockwell is being admitted to the nursing unit for diagnostic tests and treatment of essential hypertension.

A   Nursing assessment

B   Nursing interventions

C   Nursing interventions

D   Patient outcomes

E   Nursing interventions

James Rockwell:
Essential Hypertension

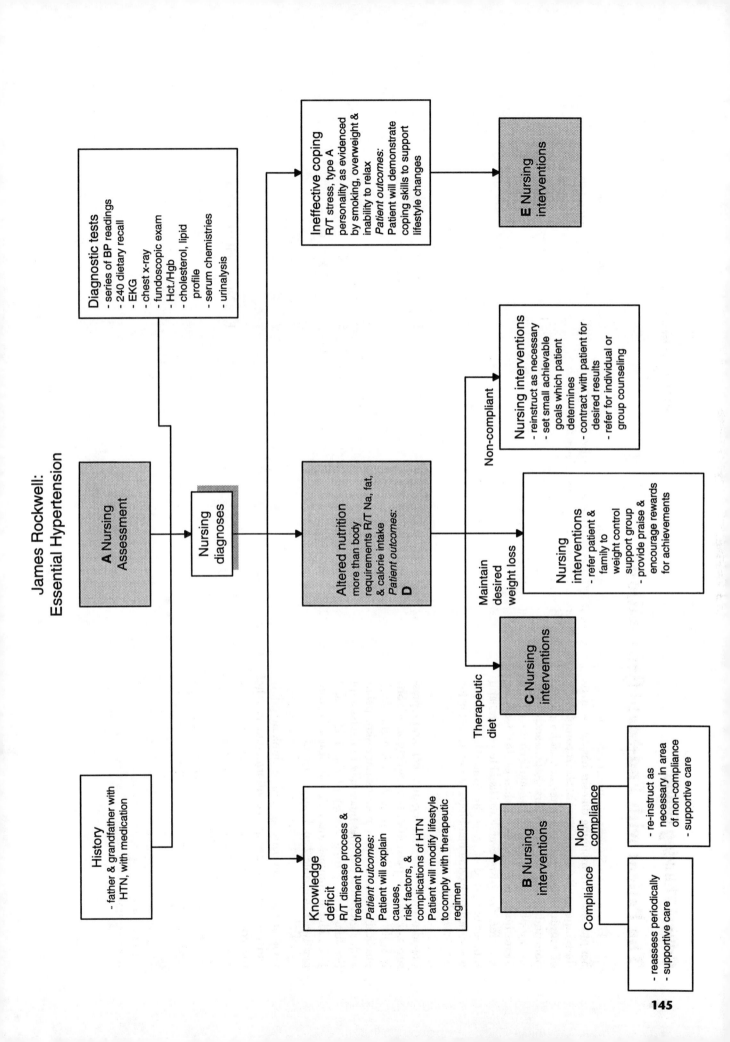

History
- father & grandfather with HTN, with medication

Diagnostic tests
- series of BP readings
- 240 dietary recall
- EKG
- chest x-ray
- fundoscopic exam
- Hct./Hgb
- cholesterol, lipid profile
- serum chemistries
- urinalysis

A Nursing Assessment

Nursing diagnoses

Ineffective coping
R/T stress, type A personality as evidenced by smoking, overweight & inability to relax
Patient outcomes:
Patient will demonstrate coping skills to support lifestyle changes

E Nursing interventions

Knowledge deficit
R/T disease process & treatment protocol
Patient outcomes:
Patient will explain causes, risk factors, & complications of HTN
Patient will modify lifestyle to comply with therapeutic regimen

B Nursing interventions

Compliance
- reassess periodically
- supportive care

Non-compliance
- re-instruct as necessary in area of non-compliance
- supportive care

Altered nutrition
more than body requirements R/T Na, fat, & calorie intake
Patient outcomes:
D

Therapeutic diet

C Nursing interventions

Maintain desired weight loss

Nursing interventions
- refer patient & family to weight control support group
- provide praise & encourage rewards for achievements

Non-compliant

Nursing interventions
- reinstruct as necessary
- set small achievable goals which patient determines
- contract with patient for desired results
- refer for individual or group counseling

Critical Thinking Guide

Name _____

The Patient with End-Stage Renal Disease

Mrs. Hurston is a 55-year-old housewife who visits her physician complaining that she has experienced flu symptoms for over a month. She is complaining of nausea, fatigue and shortness of breath on exertion, and flank pain. She wears slippers and a robe to the physician's office; she has been unable to wear shoes, tight-fitting clothes or her wedding ring for the past several weeks. Her father and brother both died of polycystic kidney disease. She is alarmed by having had blood in her urine for the past several days.

On admission to the nursing unit, her blood pressure is 192/110, pulse 108, and respiration 22. She is SOB and sleeps with two pillows at night. With physical assessment you note extreme skin pallor with a greyish color, rales bilaterally in the bases of her lungs, 3+ pitting edema of the ankles, and JVD. Her abdominal area is grossly distended, and her liver is palpable 2 to 3 finger breadths.

Look at the accompanying critical thinking guide and provide the appropriate information for the shaded boxes.

A   Nursing assessment

B   Diagnostic tests

C   Nursing interventions

D   Nursing interventions

E   Nursing interventions

Helen Hurston:
End-Stage Renal Disease

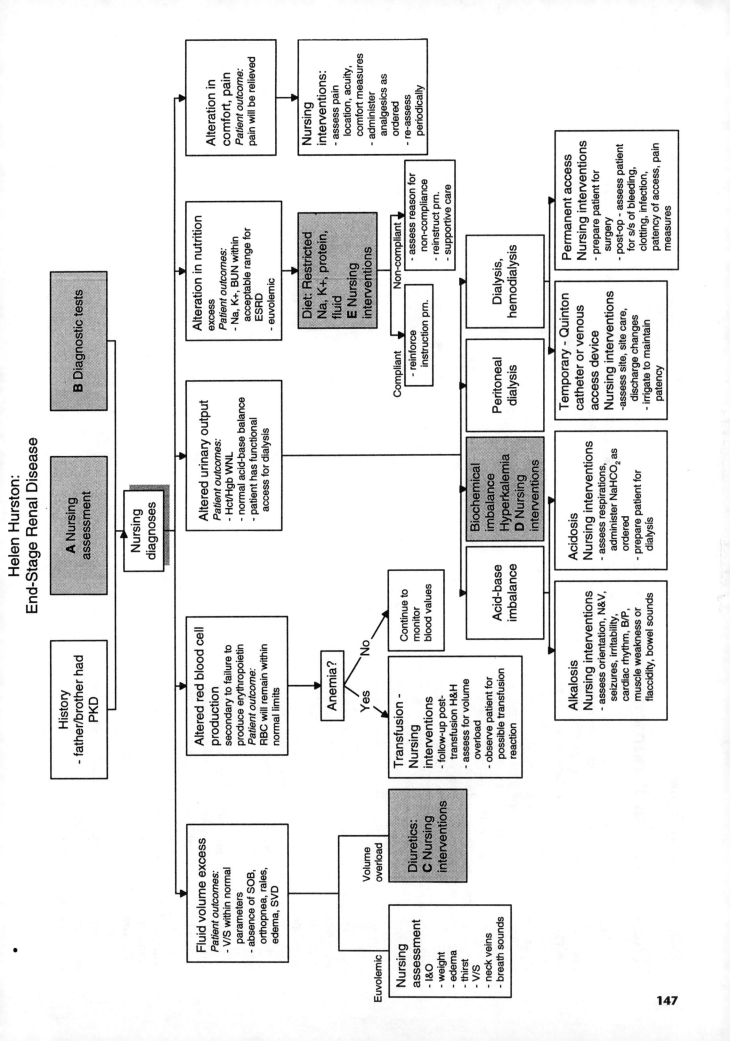

History
- father/brother had PKD

A Nursing assessment

B Diagnostic tests

Nursing diagnoses

Alteration in comfort, pain
Patient outcome: pain will be relieved

Nursing interventions:
- assess pain location, acuity, comfort measures
- administer analgesics as ordered
- re-assess periodically

Alteration in nutrition excess
Patient outcomes:
- Na, K+, BUN within acceptable range for ESRD
- euvolemic

Diet: Restricted Na, K+, protein, fluid E Nursing interventions

Non-compliant
- assess reason for non-compliance
- reinstruct prn.
- supportive care

Compliant
- reinforce instruction prn.

Altered urinary output
Patient outcomes:
- Hct/Hgb WNL
- normal acid-base balance
- patient has functional access for dialysis

Altered red blood cell production secondary to failure to produce erythropoietin
Patient outcome: RBC will remain within normal limits

Anemia?

No — Continue to monitor blood values

Yes — **Transfusion - Nursing interventions**
- follow-up post-transfusion H&H
- assess patient for volume overload
- observe patient for possible transfusion reaction

Fluid volume excess
Patient outcomes:
- V/S within normal parameters
- absence of SOB, orthopnea, rales, edema, SVD

Volume overload

Diuretics: C Nursing interventions

Euvolemic

Nursing assessment
- I&O
- weight
- edema
- thirst
- V/S
- neck veins
- breath sounds

Biochemical imbalance Hyperkalemia D Nursing interventions

Dialysis, hemodialysis

Peritoneal dialysis

Acid-base imbalance

Acidosis Nursing interventions
- assess respirations, administer NaHCO$_2$ as ordered
- prepare patient for dialysis

Alkalosis Nursing interventions
- assess orientation, N&V, seizures, irritability, cardiac rhythm, B/P, muscle weakness or flaccidity, bowel sounds

Permanent access Nursing interventions
- prepare patient for surgery
- post-op - assess patient for s/s of bleeding, clotting, infection, patency of access, pain measures

Temporary - Quinton catheter or venous access device Nursing interventions
- assess site, site care, discharge changes
- irrigate to maintain patency

147

Critical Thinking Guide

The Patient with Parkinson's Disease

Mr. Richard Smith began noticing at about age 55 that he had begun to favor the right side of his body. He unconsciously flexed his left arm while resting. When standing and walking he leaned to his right side. As he grew closer to 60 years of age, his memory was not as sharp as it used to be. He attributed these changes to aging. He once enjoyed reading more than sports, but was now unable to concentrate long enough to finish a chapter. His thinking processes slowed down; he required longer periods of time to do ordinary things such as count money, recognize that the traffic light had turned from red to green, and decide what to order for lunch.

At age 62, he notes that the trembling in his hands makes it nearly impossible to continue his employment. He also complains of urinary inconfluence, occasional constipation, and sexual dysfunction. All of these changes in body function are making him depressed. He also becomes impatient and is easily irritated. He is frightened because his mother died at age 59 of complications from Parkinson's disease.

On assessment, the nurse notes that Mr. Smith has a shuffling gait when walking. Once he is seated, his hands begin to tremble. A thorough history and physical reveal that, in addition to the above symptoms, he has a loss of postural reflexes, rigid facial expression, and an inability to walk and talk at the same time. The nurse's assessment also includes nutritional status, weight, swallowing ability, support systems, safety, equipment needs, and home environment. The neurologist diagnoses his condition as Parkinson's disease.

Look at the accompanying critical thinking guide and provide the appropriate information for the shaded boxes.

A   Physical assessment

B   Nursing interventions

C   Nursing interventions

Richard Smith:
Parkinson's Disease

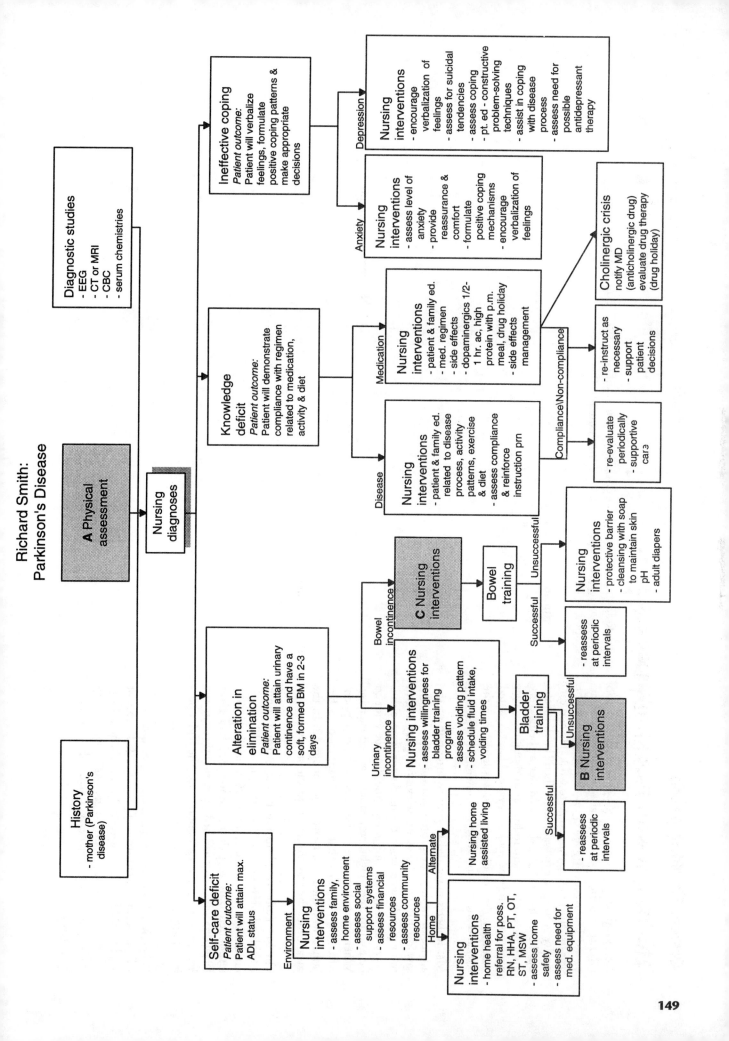

History
- mother (Parkinson's disease)

Diagnostic studies
- EEG
- CT or MRI
- CBC
- serum chemistries

A Physical assessment

Nursing diagnoses

Ineffective coping
Patient outcome: Patient will verbalize feelings, formulate positive coping patterns & make appropriate decisions

Depression

Nursing interventions
- encourage verbalization of feelings
- assess for suicidal tendencies
- assess coping
- pt. ed - constructive problem-solving techniques
- assist in coping with disease process
- assess need for possible antidepressant therapy

Anxiety

Nursing interventions
- assess level of anxiety
- provide reassurance & comfort
- formulate positive coping mechanisms
- encourage verbalization of feelings

Knowledge deficit
Patient outcome: Patient will demonstrate compliance with regimen related to medication, activity & diet

Medication

Nursing interventions
- patient & family ed.
- med. regimen
- side effects
- dopaminergics 1/2-1 hr. ac, high protein with p.m. meal, drug holiday
- side effects management

Disease

Nursing interventions
- patient & family ed. related to disease process, activity patterns, exercise & diet
- assess compliance & reinforce instruction prn

Compliance\Non-compliance

- re-instruct as necessary
- support patient decisions

- re-evaluate periodically
- supportive care

Cholinergic crisis
notify MD (anticholinergic drug)
evaluate drug therapy (drug holiday)

Alteration in elimination
Patient outcome: Patient will attain urinary continence and have a soft, formed BM in 2-3 days

Bowel incontinence

C Nursing interventions

Bowel training

Unsuccessful

Nursing interventions
- protective barrier
- cleansing with soap to maintain skin pH
- adult diapers

Successful
- reassess at periodic intervals

Urinary incontinence

Nursing interventions
- assess willingness for bladder training program
- assess voiding pattern
- schedule fluid intake, voiding times

Bladder training

Unsuccessful

B Nursing interventions

Successful
- reassess at periodic intervals

Self-care deficit
Patient outcome: Patient will attain max. ADL status

Environment

Nursing interventions
- assess family, home environment
- assess social support systems
- assess financial resources
- assess community resources

Alternate

Nursing home assisted living

Home

Nursing interventions
- home health referral for poss. RN, HHA, PT, OT, ST, MSW
- assess home safety
- assess need for med. equipment

Critical Thinking Guide

The Patient with a Cerebrovascular Accident

Look at the accompanying critical thinking guide and provide the appropriate information for the shaded boxes.

A   Nursing assessment

B   Nursing interventions

C   Nursing interventions

D   Nursing interventions

Ms. Virginia Roberts is a 58-year-old female who recently experienced a CVA at home. Her husband found her apparently asleep at the time when she was usually up preparing to go to work. He had difficulty getting her to wake up. When she did wake up, he described her as being very drowsy, unable to talk to him even though her eyes were open and she looked awake. He also stated that the right side of her mouth was lower than the left, and she was drooling.

Ms. Roberts never did pay much attention to the advice of health care professionals. From what she saw on the talk shows on television every night, most people who went to the doctor were either crazy or better off not going. She did not want to be told to lose weight, stop smoking, and exercise. When it was her time to die, it would just happen. After all, she said, that is what happened to her father, who died of a heart attack at age 48. In the meantime, she was content with the status quo.

On Ms. Robert's admission to the nursing unit, her blood pressure was 194/108, pulse 112, respirations 8 and temperature 99.8 axillary. She responded only to painful stimuli and had right facial drooping. Her nail beds were slightly cyanotic. Her right arm and leg were flaccid. She had a positive Babinski's reflex.

When Ms. Robert's physician arrives, he orders stat ABGs, serum chemistries, CBC, and CT scan of the brain. Her ABGs reveal a PO_2 of 60 and a CO_2 of 34. Just as you prepare to get Ms. Roberts onto the stretcher to go for her CT scan, she begins to have a seizure.

Virginia Roberts: Cerebrovascular Accident

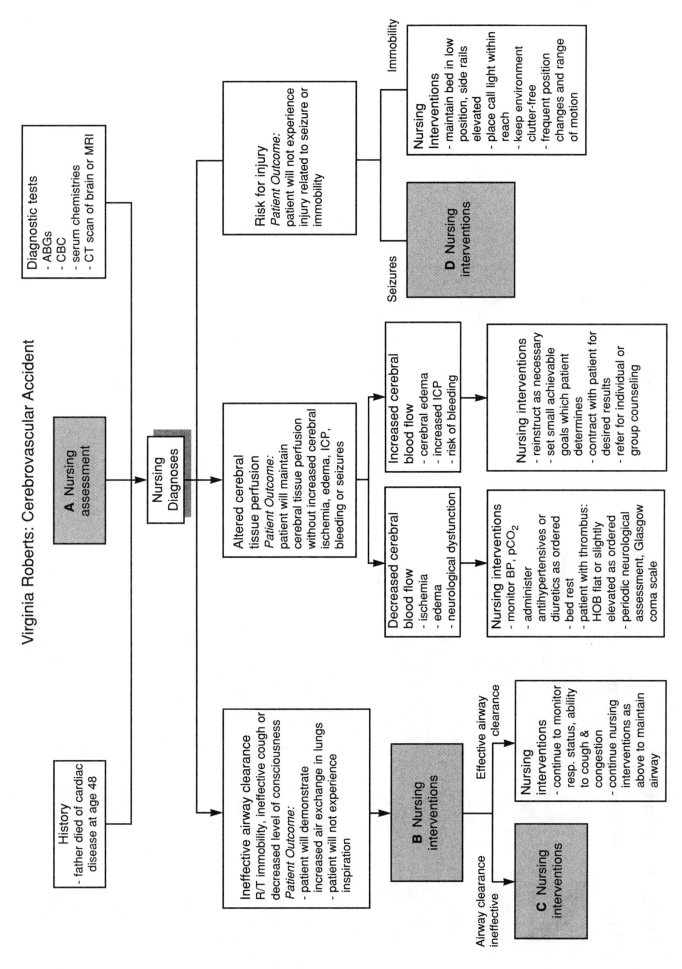

History
- father died of cardiac disease at age 48

Diagnostic tests
- ABGs
- CBC
- serum chemistries
- CT scan of brain or MRI

A Nursing assessment

Nursing Diagnoses

Risk for injury
Patient Outcome: patient will not experience injury related to seizure or immobility

Immobility

Nursing Interventions
- maintain bed in low position, side rails elevated
- place call light within reach
- keep environment clutter-free
- frequent position changes and range of motion

Seizures

D Nursing interventions

Altered cerebral tissue perfusion
Patient Outcome: patient will maintain cerebral tissue perfusion without increased cerebral ischemia, edema, ICP, bleeding or seizures

Increased cerebral blood flow
- cerebral edema
- increased ICP
- risk of bleeding

Nursing interventions
- reinstruct as necessary
- set small achievable goals which patient determines
- contract with patient for desired results
- refer for individual or group counseling

Decreased cerebral blood flow
- ischemia
- edema
- neurological dysfunction

Nursing interventions
- monitor BP, pCO_2
- administer antihypertensives or diuretics as ordered
- bed rest
- patient with thrombus: HOB flat or slightly elevated as ordered
- periodic neurological assessment, Glasgow coma scale

Ineffective airway clearance
R/T immobility, ineffective cough or decreased level of consciousness
Patient Outcome:
- patient will demonstrate increased air exchange in lungs
- patient will not experience inspiration

B Nursing interventions

Effective airway clearance

Nursing interventions
- continue to monitor resp. status, ability to cough & congestion
- continue nursing interventions as above to maintain airway

Airway clearance ineffective

C Nursing interventions

151

Critical Thinking Guide

The Patient with Glaucoma

Mr. Ricardo Gomez was admitted to the hospital emergency department after sideswiping a car. He sustained no serious injuries but stated, "I'm always bumping into things at home and now I've gone and damaged my car." Upon examination the doctor noted elevated intraocular pressure (IOP), peripheral visual field loss, and cupping of the optic disc. A risk assessment revealed a positive history of diabetes in an immediate family member (mother).

Look at the accompanying critical thinking guide and provide the appropriate information for the shaded boxes.

A   Assessment

B   Diagnostic tests

C   Emergency measures to decrease intraocular pressure

D   Assessment for visual impairment needs

E   Environmental assessment

F   Patient teaching

Ricardo Gomez: Glaucoma

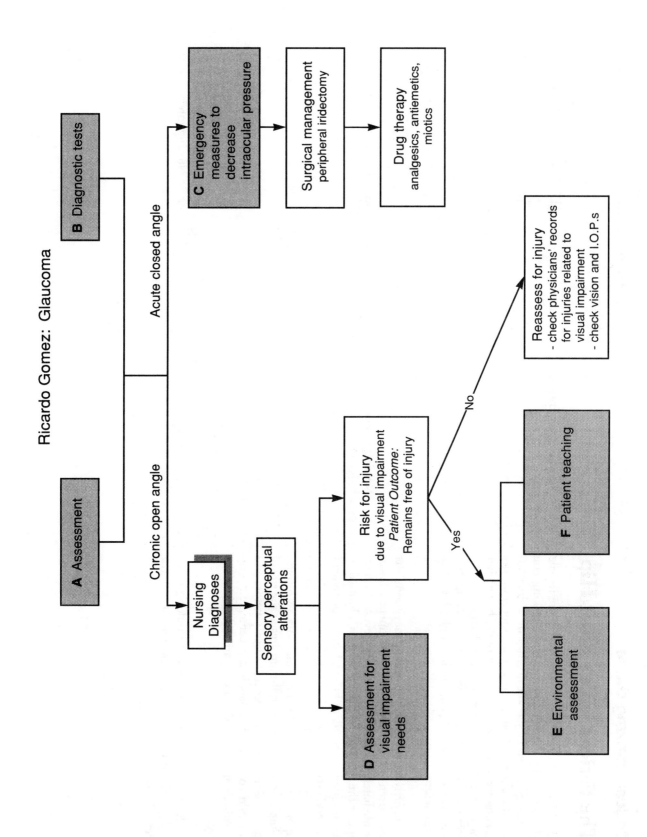

A Assessment

B Diagnostic tests

Acute closed angle

C Emergency measures to decrease intraocular pressure

Surgical management peripheral iridectomy

Drug therapy analgesics, antiemetics, miotics

Chronic open angle

Nursing Diagnoses

Sensory perceptual alterations

Risk for injury due to visual impairment
Patient Outcome:
Remains free of injury

D Assessment for visual impairment needs

No

Reassess for injury
- check physicians' records for injuries related to visual impairment
- check vision and I.O.P.s

Yes

E Environmental assessment

F Patient teaching

Critical Thinking Guide

The Patient with a Total Hip Replacement

Mrs. Elsie Whitman is a 79-year-old white female who resides in a nursing home. Upon waking one morning last week, she felt urgency of urination. When she felt she could not wait any longer for the nursing assistant to arrive, she got out of bed on her own. After standing upright, she felt dizzy. Minutes later she fell to the floor. She tried to get up, but had an excruciating pain in her right hip. She screamed for help.

Upon arriving in the hospital emergency room, she was taken to the radiology department almost immediately. X-rays of her right hip revealed a fracture at the head of the femur. She was admitted to the hospital and had right total hip replacement surgery later that day.

Upon arrival in the nursing unit, Mrs. Whitman complains of pain in the right hip area at the site of the incision. She has never had surgery before and is afraid to move. She has had a cemented joint prosthesis and is allowed only partial weight bearing.

Look at the accompanying critical thinking guide and provide the appropriate information for the shaded boxes.

A   Nursing interventions

B   Nursing interventions

C   Patient outcome

D   Patient outcome

E   Patient outcome

F   Nursing interventions

Elsie Whitman: Total Hip Replacement

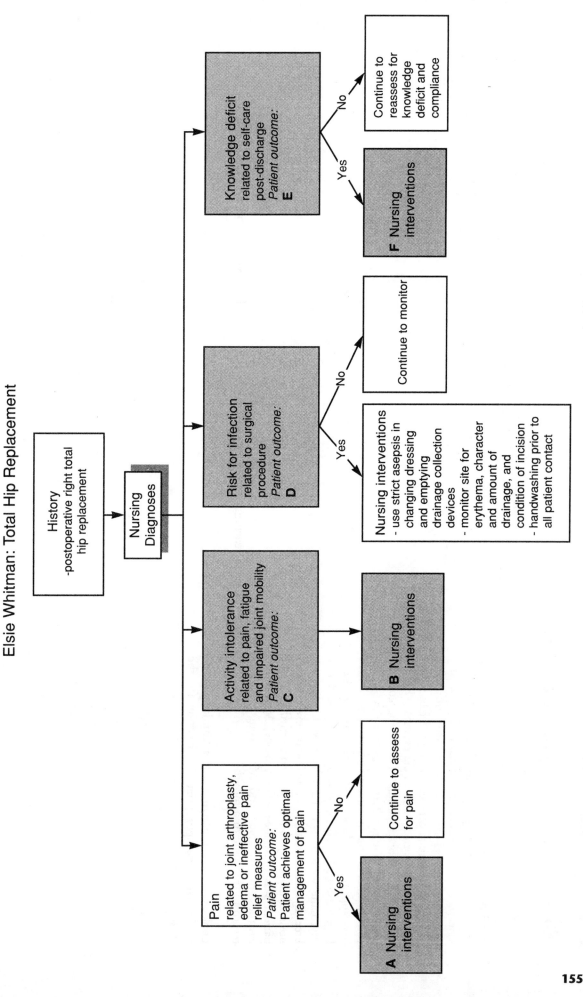

History
-postoperative right total hip replacement

Nursing Diagnoses

Pain
related to joint arthroplasty, edema or ineffective pain relief measures
Patient outcome: Patient achieves optimal management of pain

Yes → **A** Nursing interventions

No → Continue to assess for pain

Activity intolerance related to pain, fatigue and impaired joint mobility
Patient outcome:
C

B Nursing interventions

Risk for infection related to surgical procedure
Patient outcome:
D

Yes → Nursing interventions
- use strict asepsis in changing dressing and emptying drainage collection devices
- monitor site for erythema, character and amount of drainage, and condition of incision
- handwashing prior to all patient contact

No → Continue to monitor

Knowledge deficit related to self-care post-discharge
Patient outcome:
E

Yes → **F** Nursing interventions

No → Continue to reassess for knowledge deficit and compliance

Critical Thinking Guide

The Patient with Hypothyroidism

Rhonda Freeman, a 31-year-old woman, visited the clinic complaining of fatigue. She stated that her LMP was "not long ago" but could not remember the exact date. A urine pregnancy test was negative. The patient confirmed symptoms of fatigue, dry skin/hair, intolerance to cold and difficulty with mental functioning. She also stated she had symptoms of constipation and muscle cramps. Physical exam revealed bradycardia (HR = 60), and the patient stated that her lifestyle was nonathletic. She verbalized concerns over recent physical changes in her appearance. Blood pressure revealed mild hypotension, 90/56. Thyrotropin assay and free thyroxine were drawn. TSH levels were elevated. Free thyroxine estimate was below normal. A diagnosis of hypothyroidism was confirmed, and the patient was prescribed levothyroxine. Medication instruction was given and Ms Freeman was to return to the clinic in 3 months.

Look at the accompanying critical thinking guide and provide the appropriate information for the shaded boxes.

A   Nursing assessment

B   Patient teaching

C   Patient outcome

D   Nursing interventions

Rhonda Freeman:
Hypothyroidism

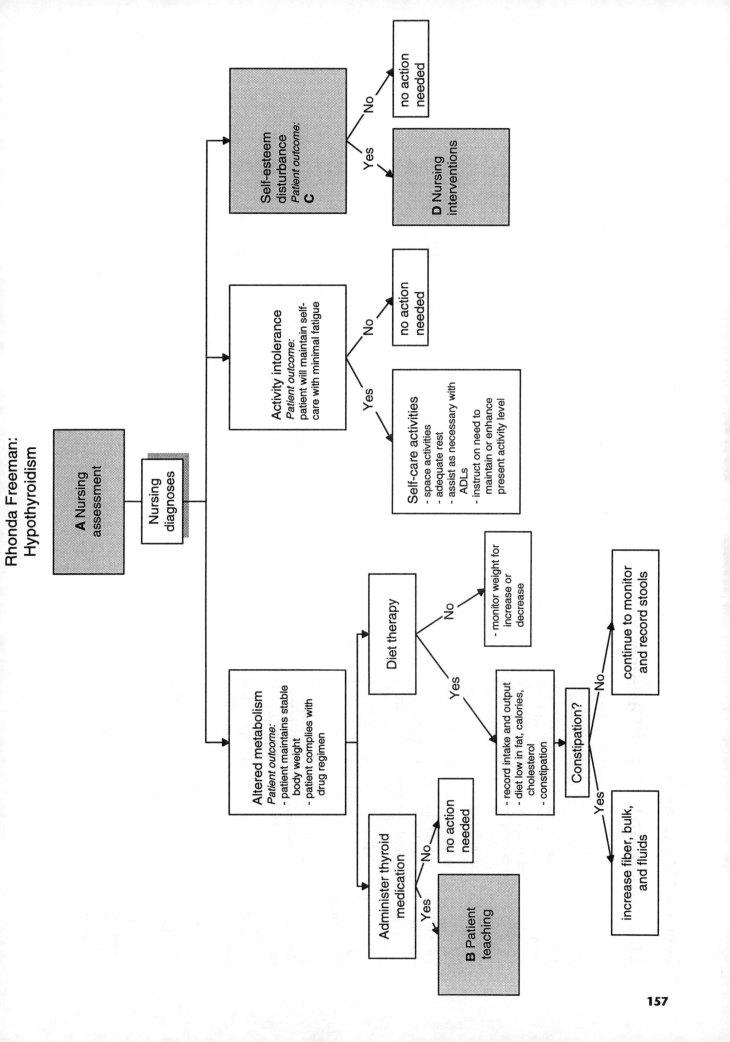

A Nursing assessment

Nursing diagnoses

Self-esteem disturbance
Patient outcome:
C

No → no action needed

Yes → **D** Nursing interventions

Activity intolerance
Patient outcome:
patient will maintain self-care with minimal fatigue

No → no action needed

Yes → **Self-care activities**
- space activities
- adequate rest
- assist as necessary with ADLs
- instruct on need to maintain or enhance present activity level

Altered metabolism
Patient outcome:
- patient maintains stable body weight
- patient complies with drug regimen

Administer thyroid medication

No → no action needed

Yes → **B** Patient teaching

Diet therapy

No → - monitor weight for increase or decrease

Yes → - record intake and output
- diet low in fat, calories, cholesterol
- constipation

Constipation?

No → continue to monitor and record stools

Yes → increase fiber, bulk, and fluids

157

Critical Thinking Guide

The Patient with Type I Diabetes Mellitus

Name _____

Joe Garcia is a 30-year-old male who has had diabetes since he was a child. Since that time his diabetes has been controlled with insulin. He also follows an 1800-calorie diabetic diet. Until this point Joe has controlled his diabetes well. He leads an active lifestyle and is compliant with his diet and medication. Joe jogs every morning before going to work. He is a paralegal at a downtown law firm and is proud of his accomplishments.

It is time for Joe's annual visit to the ophthalmologist. He is anxious about this visit as he notices his vision is not quite as clear as it once was. Since he is only 30, it is too early for him to be concerned about reading glasses. He fears he may have diabetic retinopathy. Joe visits his ophthalmologist who diagnoses his problem as such and treats it with laser therapy.

Two weeks ago, Joe was out of town at a conference. He fit jogging into his early morning preconference time, but was unable to find the indoor air-conditioned track he was accustomed to. He jogged outside the hotel and down the streets. At one point he came to road construction with loose gravel. When he got back to the hotel and took his shoes off, he noticed small pebbles in his shoes and socks. The next morning on returning from jogging, Joe noticed a bloody stain on the bottom of his sock. He inspected the bottom of his foot and found an ulcer approximately 3 cm in diameter. Joe immediately called his physician, who admitted him to the hospital for treatment of his diabetic foot ulcer.

Look at the accompanying critical thinking guide and provide the appropriate information for the shaded boxes.

A   Assessment

B   History

C   Nursing interventions

D   Nursing interventions
1. Inspection

2. Toenail care

3. Circulation

4. Bathing and socks

5. Shoes

Joe Garcia: Type I Diabetes Mellitus

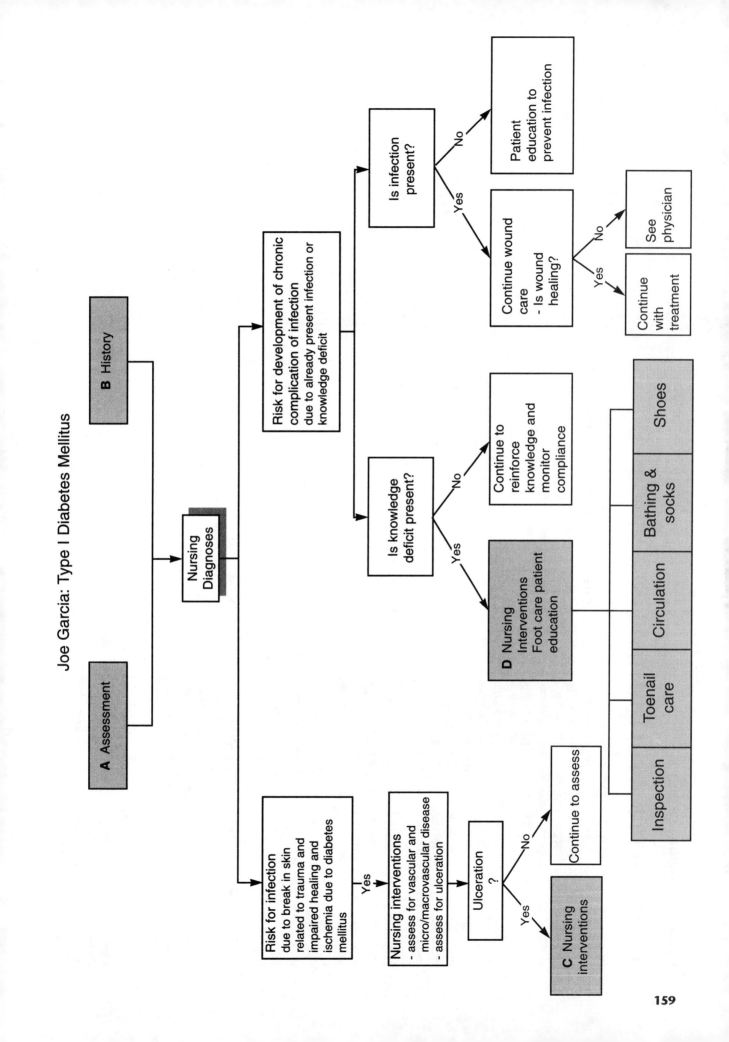

Critical Thinking Guide

The Patient with Breast Cancer and Bone Metastasis

Ms. Rachel Bernstein is a 62-year-old single, white, Jewish female. She is nulliparous and experienced menopause at age 52. Although well-educated, she has not performed breast self examinations on a routine basis. She recently had her first mammogram only because her sister insisted since she had breast cancer the previous year. Her physician had encouraged her for years, but she ignored him because she felt this unnecessary at her age. Besides, she didn't feel a mammogram would be effective since she has had fibrocystic breast disease since she was a teenager. She thought women her age who had never married just didn't get breast cancer.

Her mammogram revealed several tumors 5 to 10 cm in diameter bilaterally throughout her breasts. The radiologist suspected she also had lymph node involvement and instructed her to visit her physician and as soon as possible for biopsy. Outpatient surgery for biopsies revealed diffuse carcinoma throughout both breasts and involving the lymph system. She was then scheduled for a bilateral radical mastectomy.

Following her mastectomies, she anticipated radiation and/or chemotherapy. However, it was determined through a bone scan that she had bone metastasis. What she had attributed to arthritic pain for the previous months was actually cancer of the bone.

You receive Ms. Bernstein postop from the postanesthesia care unit. She is awake and complaining of mild discomfort related to her surgery. She feels for her bandages and asks the nurse what her chest looks like now.

Look at the accompanying critical thinking guide and provide the appropriate information for the shaded boxes.

A Nursing assessment

B Diagnostic studies

C Nursing interventions

D Nursing interventions

E Patient outcome

F Nursing interventions

G Nursing interventions

Rachel Bernstein: Breast Cancer

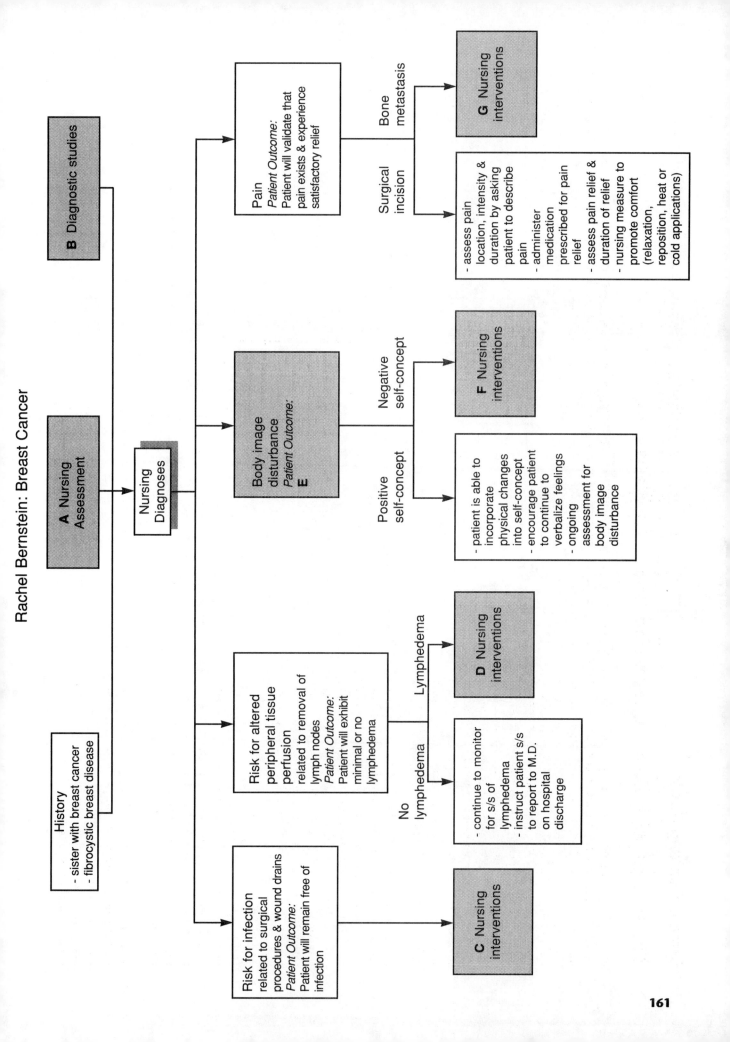

A Nursing Assessment

History
- sister with breast cancer
- fibrocystic breast disease

B Diagnostic studies

Nursing Diagnoses

Risk for infection related to surgical procedures & wound drains
Patient Outcome: Patient will remain free of infection

C Nursing interventions

Risk for altered peripheral tissue perfusion related to removal of lymph nodes
Patient Outcome: Patient will exhibit minimal or no lymphedema

No lymphedema
- continue to monitor for s/s of lymphedema
- instruct patient s/s to report to M.D. on hospital discharge

Lymphedema

D Nursing interventions

Body image disturbance
Patient Outcome:
E

Positive self-concept
- patient is able to incorporate physical changes into self-concept
- encourage patient to continue to verbalize feelings
- ongoing assessment for body image disturbance

Negative self-concept

F Nursing interventions

Pain
Patient Outcome: Patient will validate that pain exists & experience satisfactory relief

Surgical incision
- assess pain location, intensity & duration by asking patient to describe pain
- administer medication prescribed for pain relief
- assess pain relief & duration of relief
- nursing measure to promote comfort (relaxation, reposition, heat or cold applications)

Bone metastasis

G Nursing interventions

161